Seventh Heaven

www.booksattransworld.co.uk

Seventh Heaven

A TOTALLY NEW AND ENLIGHTENING VISION OF SEXUALITY

Linda Sonntag

BANTAM BOOKS

LONDON • TORONTO • SYDNEY • AUCKLAND • JOHANNESBURG

SEVENTH HEAVEN
A BANTAM BOOK: 0 553 81624 1

First publication in Great Britain

PRINTING HISTORY
Bantam edition published 2005

1 3 5 7 9 10 8 6 4 2

Set in 11/18pt Nofret by
Falcon Oast Graphic Art Ltd.

Bantam Books are published by Transworld Publishers,
61–63 Uxbridge Road, London W5 5SA,
a division of The Random House Group Ltd,
in Australia by Random House Australia (Pty) Ltd,
20 Alfred Street, Milsons Point, Sydney, NSW 2061, Australia,
in New Zealand by Random House New Zealand Ltd,
18 Poland Road, Glenfield, Auckland 10, New Zealand
and in South Africa by Random House (Pty) Ltd,
Endulini, 5a Jubilee Road, Parktown 2193, South Africa.

Printed and bound in Great Britain by
Mackays of Chatham plc, Chatham, Kent

Papers used by Transworld Publishers are natural, recyclable products
made from wood grown in sustainable forests. The manufacturing
processes conform to the environmental regulations of the
country of origin.

Contents

*The thrill of the erotic lies
in the shadows, in the
glimpse of a bare arm, the
curve of a shoulder, a
damp curl of hair at the
nape of the neck.*

INTRODUCTION

The Seven Scrolls

EROTICISM IS ELUSIVE. IT UNFOLDS IN AN inner life of strong feelings and vivid fantasies; it blooms in a suspended reality that is close to trance, when a secret hint or a veiled promise sparks the imagination and inflames desire. The thrill of the erotic lies in the shadows, in the glimpse of a bare arm, the curve of a shoulder, a damp curl of hair at the nape of the neck. It cannot be evoked by the punchy instructional style of modern guides that present sex as a set of techniques unclouded by emotion, stripping it of all its mystery and its relevance to life.

The approach of the ancients was more subtle

and more profound. The mystics of India aimed to invoke and experience the truth of the erotic with all their senses, combining words with symbols, scents, sounds and colours to heighten the sacred-ness of touch in sexual ritual. The Chinese revered the delights of sex as a path to health and longevity. They made a detailed and sensitive study of erotic arousal and sexual response five millennia before Western scientists put sex under the microscope in their laboratories. And all over the world, the ancients used sexuality, the most intense and beautiful of sensual experiences, to intuit the Divine.

This book aims to refine our experience of the erotic in the light of lost sexual wisdom, to intensify the pleasure and understanding between couples, improving relationships in and out of bed.

Seventh Heaven follows the format of the ancient Chinese pillow books, in which the Yellow Emperor consulted three of his favourite concubines on sexual matters both practical and emotional. In this book a modern couple, Adam and Eve, discuss all aspects of erotic love with three courtesans: from India, France and Japan.

The three experts answer questions both trivial and profound, inspiring Adam and Eve with their insights and detailed imaginative advice. The wealth of ancient sexual wisdom the courtesans bring from their own traditions and from around the world contains secrets that cannot be communicated in a few words. While they are subtle, these secrets are also powerful enough to transform the love life of Adam and Eve and transport them to the sensual bliss of the Seventh Heaven.

❦

Seventh Heaven takes the form of seven scrolls. These scrolls of faded parchment caught Adam's eye one day as he was browsing through a second-hand bookshop looking for an erotic gift for Eve. That night in bed, as she lay next to him, he began to

read from the first scroll, with delightfully
unexpected consequences ...

SCROLL ONE

The Gateway to Heaven

❧

The Courtesans' Parchment

The essence of Tantra is an attitude of complete awareness and openness to experience, both sexual and spiritual.

EX LIES AT THE VERY HEART OF CULTURE in the East. For thousands of years it has been treasured as a source of sensual pleasure that satisfies the body and the soul, bringing health and vitality and offering a route to spiritual bliss. In the East sex has always been deeply connected with religion, for sex and religion are the twin paths to immortality. Religion offers spiritual enlightenment; through sex the bloodline is everlastingly continued into future generations, and erotic ecstasy unites the two paths, giving a sense of heaven on earth. Because sex and religion were at one in the ancient world, there was no prudery or repression, but an open and practical attitude towards investigating how to improve erotic experience.

About five thousand years ago the mountains of Tibet and Nepal witnessed the birth of a movement called Tantra, whose followers dedicated themselves to the study of sex as religion. The basic principle of Tantra was that women possess more spiritual energy and sexual stamina than men, who become sexually exhausted relatively quickly. The aim of Tantra was to find ways of prolonging sexual activity without exhaustion. By close observation of their own arousal, together with meditation, and yogic exercises that combined the physical and the spiritual, the Tantrics discovered how to control and refine their sexual response so that men could delay ejaculation, and both men and women could become multi-orgasmic.

Tantra has always been viewed with particular suspicion in the West because of its association with spells and magic ritual. Not only that – when a Westerner thinks of Tantra the image that comes to mind is one of a couple entwined in an impossibly contorted pose, staring without motion or emotion into one another's eyes. But there is much more to Tantra than that.

The essence of Tantra is an attitude of complete awareness and openness to experience, both sexual and spiritual. The couple in the impossible position were not meant to be real-life lovers but gods, usually Shiva, the Lord of Yoga, and his heavenly concubines, or royal princes flatteringly depicted as gods. The delightful miniatures in which they appear are symbolic of that moment of ecstatic stillness at the heart of the turmoil of sexual passion that the Tantrics learned to hold onto, transforming ejaculation into orgasm. They did indeed teach their students to slow down their lovemaking and hold poses for seconds or even minutes on end. The point of this exercise was to increase their awareness of each and every sensation in the body, because only by knowing and understanding our sexuality can we begin to harness its energy and exercise some control over the way we experience pleasure.

The Tantric attitude of open curiosity and reverence towards sex strongly influenced the religions and philosophies of the two vast countries on either side of the Himalayas into which it flowed. In India, both Buddhism and Hinduism have Tantric sects, but they are disavowed by the mainstream and called the 'left-hand path' for their association with the dark arts and their willingness to experiment with every kind of sensation. For the Tantrics, sex has little to do with morality.

In China, the principles of Tantric sex were incorporated into the worldview called the Tao, or 'the Way'. At the heart of Taoism lies the very simple idea of a universal life force or energy called *chi*. The aim of Taoism is to maximize the flow of chi in the body and to use its transformational power for physical and spiritual health. The way to maximize the flow of chi is to balance the two opposing principles that create chi, passive *yin* and active *yang.* Since yin and yang are the female and male poles of the sexual spectrum that exist within all of us, one of the major ways of bringing them into harmony is through sex.

The Taoist tradition of sexual wisdom was handed down from the time of the Yellow Emperor, Huang–Di, who reigned in the third millennium BCE, and first put into writing around two thousand three hundred years ago in the world's earliest sex manuals. These books take the form of conversations between the Yellow Emperor and three courtesans, the Essential Girl, the Mysterious Girl and the Rainbow Girl, who in their role as advisers became the world's first sex therapists. Their pupil is occasionally petulant and despairing of his efforts in the imperial bedchamber, but he confronts his problems with openness and honesty. 'Sometimes I want to make love,' he complains, 'yet my Jade Stalk will not rise up. My face betrays my shame and my perspiration drops like pearls. My heart and my sentiments are fired by lust, but I have to help with my fingers. How can I be strong?'

The three courtesans teach the Emperor the secrets of preparing his mind and body for sex; they help him navigate the tumultuous seas of a woman's emotions and understand the complexities of her sexual response. Their acute observations of erotic arousal educated Chinese lovers for more than two millennia before such detailed knowledge was available in the West.

It is a common misunderstanding that the Tao of sex regards women as passive and men as active. This is far from the truth. The three courtesans explain that woman is the source of the nourishing yin qualities of stability and continuity, an inexhaustible powerhouse of vitality and sexual energy. They compare her ability to enjoy making love for hours on end with the male tendency to ejaculate within minutes. 'The male is easily aroused but quick to retreat,' they point out. 'The female is slow to be aroused and slow to be satiated.' The courtesans call female orgasm by the poetic name of 'high tide', for a woman's sexuality is like the sea, it swells and peaks, falls and rises again, a force of nature that cannot be spent or diminished. But when a man ejaculates they say he has 'lost his essence', 'thrown it away' or 'surrendered'. The lost essence is not just the semen, but the energy that goes with it.

The Taoists knew that this fundamental in-equality of the sexes lies at the root of all the problems of the bedroom and spills over into everyday life to cause dissatisfaction and resent-ment between men and women. They concluded that a good relationship – and harmony and happiness in the home – depended on a man learn-ing how to satisfy his lover in bed. And since ejaculation was likely to end the sexual encounter before the woman was satisfied, the Taoists aimed to teach men how to delay and even withhold ejaculation so that women could experience as much caressing and as many orgasms as they wished.

Hearing this, the Yellow Emperor is immediately alarmed – as any man might be – wondering how he can experience true pleasure in sex without ejaculating. If by learning the secrets of the Tao he ejaculates less and less, he asks, won't his pleasure diminish accordingly? The answer is: not at all! In fact, pleasure will immeasurably increase. After ejaculating, a man feels exhausted, his ears may start to buzz, his eyelids droop, and he longs for sleep. His limbs ache and he feels weak and thirsty – his ejaculation was a brief moment of bliss followed by hours of weariness. 'This is not true pleasure!' exclaim the courtesans.

However, if a man learns how to retain his semen so he can prolong lovemaking, and occasionally denies himself the fleeting delight of ejaculation altogether, his body will grow strong, his mind will be clear, and his vision and hearing will improve. Moreover, his love for his woman, his lust and his vitality will greatly increase. He will feel as if he could never get enough of her. 'Is that not the true and lasting pleasure of sex?' they ask.

The Taoists knew that a man who retains high levels of hormones and semen by learning ejaculation control experiences a greatly improved appetite for sex, with more energy and stamina. Sex lasts longer and makes him feel younger, instead of wearing him out. And the surprising thing is that as he learns to withhold ejaculation, he will discover that this does not mean robbing himself of orgasm, because orgasm and ejaculation, as the Chinese knew five thousand years ago and the West discovered only recently, are entirely separate phenomena. And the more he practises withholding, the stronger orgasms he will have, without ejaculating, until the sensation spreads like wave after wave radiating from his genitals to flood his whole body.

While the Emperor enthusiastically practises simple exercises in muscle and breath control that will help him delay his ejaculation, the courtesans teach him a code of behaviour for use in and out of the bedroom that will harmonize relations with his beloved. This system is called the Five Virtues and it has just as much relevance to both sexes today as it did then.

The first virtue of sex is *benevolence*, which means tenderness, generosity and selflessness. The second is *justice*. Neither party should ever force sex on the other, or even persuade the other to have sex when he or she is not in the mood, for no good will come from it. The third virtue is *courtesy*. In the arena of sex this means tact, mutual respect, and reverence for the sex act itself. A man should always hold back to give his partner the time and opportunity to experience pleasure to the full. The fourth virtue of sex is *honesty*. The Tao calls for an open attitude of sharing, truthfulness about one's feelings, and objectivity about one's ability to satisfy one's partner. It recognizes that talking about sex and about feelings can bring a couple closer together and open up their sex life to be richer and more rewarding. Finally, the fifth virtue of sex is *wisdom*.

This simply means using common sense, kindness and intuition in discovering how to please your partner.

The Chinese produced pillow books that were both pragmatic in their advice and beautifully illustrated. They were intended as bedtime reading for men and women, and especially for the initiation of young brides. It was the custom in ancient China for a man to marry at around thirty-six and to take a bride a third his age. On their wedding night he would sit her on his knee and show her the book, talking softly to her and beginning a gentle exploration of her body that might take several nights. At last, when the bride's sexual awakening was complete, her confidence and her desire aroused, she demanded to experience for herself all that she had been shown and told. And it was easy for her to put her desire into words because the language of the pillow books was delightfully poetic, at once familiar and picturesque, designed for sensuality. The penis could be called the Jade Stalk, the Red Bird, the Heavenly Dragon Pillar or the Swelling Mushroom. The vulva was the Open Peony Blossom or the Golden Lotus; the vagina the Golden Vase. So different from the crude terminology common in the West today that makes it difficult to speak of sex with tenderness.

After the Taoists came the Confucians and with them an era of sexual repression in which many of the beautifully decorated pillow books were destroyed and much of the wisdom they contained was lost or forgotten. But fragments of Taoist sexual writings were smuggled out of China into Japan and across the mountains to India, where in the third century CE their sophisticated approach probably influenced Vatsyayana Mallanaga, the writer of the most famous of ancient pillow books, the *Kamasutra*.

Addressed to a wealthy elite, this treatise on the science of love describes techniques of courting and seduction against a background steaming with adultery, intrigue and betrayal. In Indian mythology Kama is the god of love, and like Eros and Cupid he is an archer. Kama draws a bow made of sugar strung with bees. In his quiver are five arrows, each tipped with the essence of a different flower to be aimed at one of the five senses. The *Kamasutra* is pierced through with love's phallic arrow, the symbol of love as desire, lust and sex. Kama is everything that delights the senses – especially the male senses:

> *Kama is pleasure, and its limbs are*
> *jewellery, perfumed oils and garlands,*
> *as well as forest groves, rooftop gardens,*
> *the playing of lutes and wine.*
> *Its base is women – unrestrained, beautiful, young,*
> *amorous, flirtatious, clever at flattery,*
> *drawing to themselves the minds and hearts of men.*

> Yashodhara Indrapada, 13th century

The charm of the *Kamasutra* lies in its exotic evocation of a life dedicated to sensuality. The pleasure quarters of Vatsyayana's model citizen comprised an inner room, the private domain of his wives, and an outer room with a soft bed covered with a clean white counterpane. There were pillows at either end of the bed, and above it a canopy decorated with garlands of flowers. The air was heady with rich perfumes. Beside the bed was a couch and next to it a low table on which were arranged fragrant ointments and dishes of scented bark and seeds that were chewed to sweeten the breath. The habit of chewing mildly anaesthetic betel nuts, which produces an excess of pink saliva, necessitated the discreet presence of a spittoon. Also to hand were various trinkets and games: a box of ornaments, a lute hanging from a peg made of an elephant's tusk, a drawing board, story books, board games and dice for gambling. Vatsyayana knew that if lovers played together out of bed they would be more playful in bed, so he recommended entertainments of all kinds for fun and relaxation.

Outside the playroom, a terrace overlooked a beautiful garden. On hot sultry nights the women of the harem would spread rugs and cushions under the stars and prepare to make love to the sound of a chorus of crickets and frogs. In the garden the citizen had installed soothing water features, cages of singing birds, a bower covered in creepers and a workshop equipped for diversions such as carving and spinning. Rigged up here and there among the trees were hammocks and various types of swing that could be moved up and down as well as back and forth. Swings were often used during lovemaking, particularly when the citizen entertained several of his wives at once.

On rising, the student of the *Kamasutra* performed an elaborate toilette, which included shaving all body hair, bathing, perfuming his body and making up his eyes in front of a mirror. He would chew betel leaves to freshen his breath, perhaps stain his teeth red or black, then take breakfast, after which he spent some time training his parrots to speak and his quails, cocks and rams to fight. The remaining hour or two before lunch were devoted to literature and drama. A nap followed during the heat of the day. Then the citizen dressed in his finery and ornaments and went out visiting. Sitting with friends, he would talk and drink cordials made from the bark of trees, as well as from fruits and flowers. Other social diversions included picnics, boating parties, singing, walking in the garden and pelting one another with the scented blossoms of the kadamba tree. Sometimes there were swimming parties, with the servants instructed to make sure that no dangerous animals lurked in the water. All this was a gentle build-up to the pleasures of the night. When dusk fell, the men waited in a room full of perfume and flowers for the women of their choice to arrive.

The *Kamasutra* recommends several ways of wooing. When a man loves a girl he should sit next to her at parties and take every opportunity to touch her. Gently he places his foot upon hers and touches each of her toes with his own, pressing down significantly on the ends of her nails. If he is a visitor in her house and she is washing his feet, he squeezes one of her fingers between two of his toes, and whenever their eyes meet he looks at her with longing. As she begins to fall in love with him, he craftily feigns illness and begs her to come to his house. There she finds him lounging on a couch in a darkened room; he presses her cool hand on his forehead, moaning that only she can administer the medicine that will cure him. He persuades her to tend him with herbal remedies for three days and nights, all the while talking to her softly, letting her into the secrets of his heart. Vatsya notes that even though a man truly loves a woman, he will never be able to win her over without a great deal of talk.

In charming a woman with romantic conversation, the citizen is advised to show 'an increased liking for the new foliage of trees and such things'. If his sweet words fall on deaf ears, he should surreptitiously feed her with some intoxicating substance, carry her off and enjoy her before she has time to come round, then immediately set up the marriage ceremony. Alternatively, he can ambush the reluctant woman while she is walking in the garden, attack and kill her guards, then carry her off and proceed as before. Vatsyayana considered sexual harassment, drugging, murder and rape to be quite acceptable. If a woman said no, he would encourage a man to read in her eyes that she meant yes. He urges his reader to disregard women's protests, or to take them as encouragement.

A married woman needs a different approach. Poetic talk of budding leaves will be wasted here. Instead, the citizen should adopt the discreet language of amorous signs: pull on his moustache, make a clicking sound with his fingernails, cause his ornaments to tinkle and bite his lower lip. His object in seducing a married woman may not be lust after all, but a burning desire to destroy her husband. Once she has been won over, the humiliated husband can be killed with relish and robbed of his money and possessions.

Adultery was a popular pastime in ancient India, and daily life offered plenty of opportunity for adventure. The man who delivered corn and filled the householder's granary was invited indoors by his wife, as were the handyman, the cleaner, the labourer in the fields and the door–to–door salesmen of cotton, wool, flax and hemp. While the cowherds enjoyed the cowgirls, the superintendents of widows enjoyed the widows in their charge and the superintendents of markets found secret corners in which to entertain their female customers. On warm evenings villagers roamed the streets looking for excitement; those left at home bedded the wives of their sons.

The status of a wife was poor. Vatsyayana declares that a man is justified in taking a second wife if his first is ill-tempered, if she produces no children, or only daughters, or merely if he has a roving eye. For this reason, he advises the wife to work very hard to secure the heart of her husband and master the arts of the Kama Shastra, a sort of finishing school syllabus for upper-class wives. In addition to the traditional female accomplishments of singing, dancing and drawing, the Kama Shastra taught more unusual skills. These included sorcery, sword-fighting and the knowledge of poisons. If a second wife is chosen despite all her efforts to please, the first wife has to become even more subservient, doing all she can to excel in self-denial (perhaps nourishing the thought that if things get too bad, she can call on her expertise in the dark arts to vanquish her rival).

In this world of formalized behaviour, problems – that is, women's problems due to ill-treatment by their husbands – must be driven underground. Wives must learn to bite their lip. If a husband behaves badly, his wife should not blame him, even if he has beaten her. She should avoid black looks, talking behind his back, and standing around in doorways where people can see and admire her. Above all, she should not take revenge by wandering in pleasure groves, where there is certain danger of meeting attractive men with time on their hands. Instead, she should remain dutifully indoors, keeping her body, her teeth, her hair and everything belonging to her tidy, sweet and clean.

Should a love quarrel erupt despite the woman's best efforts to grit her perfectly clean teeth and avoid marring her beauty with murderous looks, it must follow a prescribed pattern. The wife is allowed to pull her husband's hair and kick him, but she should withdraw no further than the doorway. Aggressive feelings are to be contained in ritual striking, crying out, biting, and piercing with the nails. In fact, Vatsyayana considers violence and sadism a normal part of life. He gives lists prescribing with what force and on which parts of the body cruel practices may be carried out.

Perhaps boredom as well as the suppression of women led men of the indolent upper classes into sadistic practices, for violence between lovers was recommended in passion as well as in anger. Needless to say, most of it was directed at the female sex. Nails could be pressed into the lover's armpits, throat, breasts, lips, midriff, buttocks and thighs, leaving bruises like half-moons, the tracks of a hare or the leaf of a blue lotus; sometimes they appeared to have been made by a peacock's foot or a tiger's claw. Vatsyayana reckoned that such marks were worn with pride by women on their bare breasts so that when they wandered through the pleasure gardens they would inflame the heart of any man who passed. He favoured strong pointed nails and strong teeth that would take well to dyeing. He liked to see them even, unbroken and, above all, sharp. Good teeth could be used to inflict various bites on the lover's skin, which were given names, such as the hidden bite, the swollen bite, the line of jewels, the broken cloud and the bite of the boar.

Courtesans and nuns were the only women who could move freely in society in ancient India. While other women, both single and married, are seen as ripe fruits to be plucked for male enjoyment, Vatsyayana treats courtesans as the equals of men, giving them the same sort of advice he gives to men about tricking the opposite sex. If her lover is not generous, he suggests twenty-seven ways in which a clever courtesan can persuade him to part with cash and jewels. For instance, she can break down in tears and sob that she is destitute because she has been robbed or her house has burned down. She can plead for cash to buy new clothes or upgrade her cooking utensils in line with those of her friends. Or she can simply make him jealous by telling him how lavishly his rivals treat her.

When a woman wants to make a man fall in love with her, the first thing is not to appear too eager, says Vatsya, because men are likely to despise things that are too easily acquired. Instead of visiting the man she has set her sights on, a woman should employ her servants to discover his state of mind. She may send her jesters, masseurs and confidantes to entertain and beguile him. On their return, she will question them closely, and if she likes what she hears, she will invite the man to watch a battle between her fighting cocks. Then she can give him a well chosen present, something especially designed to arouse his curiosity and inspire intimate regard. And she can captivate his imagination by telling him intriguing stories. To ensure that he doesn't forget her after the visit, she will send her female attendant to his house from time to time, to bring him witty and mischievous messages and small amusing gifts. In this way, he will soon be won over.

And once he is won, the way to keep him is to treat him like a god. The courtesan was a highly skilled manipulator of male vanity. Socially and intellectually at least the equal of her lover, her job was to make him feel that, nevertheless, she was his slave. Vatsya gives detailed instructions for flatter–ing the male ego. He comes up with some ingenious ideas. A woman should send her servant to the man's house to fetch the flowers his gardener arranged for him the day before, so that she can take pleasure in what he has already enjoyed. When she is with him, she should present a perfect mirror to his feelings, laughing when he is happy, pining away when he is sick, looking downcast even when he sighs or yawns. She vows hatred of his enemies, wishes fervently to have a child by him, and delights in eating the scraps from his plate. She pleasures him in any way he wants and, of course, expresses amazement at his accomplishments and his rare knowledge of the sexual arts. If anyone tries to come between them, she threatens to take her own life by poisoning, stabbing or hanging.

The exclusive and highly skilled courtesan of ancient India was called a *ganika*. Her status was far above that of the humble prostitute, the *mahanagni*, literally 'she of great nakedness', a woman who bared herself to many men. Above the *mahanagni* were many ranks of actresses, and the harem also had its own hierarchy. Inside the palace walls there were girls who carried pitchers, garlands, jewellery, ornaments, fans or jars of perfumed water. There were girls who waited in attendance at the throne, or who walked in procession by the king, such as his royal umbrella–bearer. There were others in charge of bathing or dressing his royal personage. But all these were *odalisques*, or slaves.

Only the accomplished and independent *ganika* could make her fortune as the mistress of one very wealthy man. If she was young, exceptionally beautiful and outstandingly talented and witty, she could name her price and be patronized by poets and orators, ministers of state, and the most elevated aristocrats; she could even tempt the king to desert his harem to spend a night in her company. He would send a thousand gold coins and a chest full of jewels to secure her services in advance. The richest courtesans owned land and property and invested money in philanthropic projects, such as sinking wells, building bridges, feeding the poor and laying out gardens and groves of mangoes around Buddhist temples and monasteries.

❧

Even more mysterious than the voluptuous Indian courtesan is the geisha, the most elusive erotic icon of the East. Part actress, part sorceress, this creature of the night inhabits the glittering *demi-monde*, weaving her spells in a realm of dreams. Her name, *geisha*, means artist; the subject of her art is herself. Everything she creates and does, from her appearance to her manners and the way she sits, walks and speaks, is polished into an artwork of cultivated elegance and mystique.

The geisha has always stood apart from even the most sought-after courtesan because while men can buy her company at a banquet or a party, or for a trip to the theatre or a private supper, her sexual favours are not on offer. Men have ruined themselves in pursuit of these most brilliant, witty and sophisticated of women, and still been rejected. The geisha may be the mistress of a wealthy and powerful man, and her patron may give her generous gifts and a handsome allowance that more than covers the cost of her fabulously expensive wardrobe. But still she prefers to retain her independence and live in the geisha house among her adopted mothers and sisters, because her work is both her pleasure and her life.

A geisha may form a lifelong intimate relationship with her protector, but she always remains outside the marriage market. In Japan marriage is traditionally a social and economic institution with carefully arranged matches and early motherhood. Society has always looked askance at any other option for a woman. Until recently, wives had little freedom and no economic independence and girls were not brought up to be equal to men in conversation. Though the geisha stood apart from society, her role was accepted; indeed the wife of a wealthy man would expect her husband to take a geisha mistress as a mark of his high status – even inviting her to their home to entertain their guests. Likewise, respectable mothers sent their sons to the teahouses to be educated by geishas in the art of conversation. Some may have learned other things too, for the geisha and her lovers made a detailed study of the ancient Chinese pillow books that had been smuggled into Japan.

The geisha profession dates from the seventeenth century when plans were drawn up to build the city of Edo, now Tokyo, and the pleasure quarter was laid out before everything else. The first geishas were actually men, actors of the *kabuki* theatre, who sang and danced in the teahouses, told jokes and amusing anecdotes and sold sexual favours. By the middle of the eighteenth century the pleasure quarter was known by the poetic name of the Floating World, a world of illusion as transient as the tumbling cherry blossoms, a place where men could give themselves over to the pursuit of pleasure and forget everyday reality. It was a world of paper lanterns and music, full of laughter and the scent of jasmine, a world of glamour, frivolity and decadent display. Rebels and outcasts took refuge there and writers and painters of erotica found freedom and inspiration.

The Nightless City of the pleasure quarter was honeycombed with waterways and canals and the water lapped at the terraces of the teahouses. The geishas were part of the 'water trade', for water is the feminine element and encompasses women, sexuality, love, and drinking at out-of-hours bars, all specialities of the Floating World. At its height, the water trade boasted three thousand elegantly dressed and fantastically coiffed geishas, who were said to bloom in rivalry like primroses in the grass. For those who could not afford their company there were courtesans and prostitutes of many ranks and subdivisions. Ladies of pleasure erected tents along the riverbank, where 'pillow service', laundry and mending could be booked by the month. The prostitutes of Edo were said to know forty-eight or even fifty-five different positions for lovemaking, and a man could tell their skill by the way their pubic hair was plucked and clipped and the aphrodisiacs and sex toys that they offered him. But most men visited the Floating World for pleasures more elusive than mere sexual intercourse – to immerse themselves in erotic fantasy and dreams.

The geisha was an icon of fashion, the epitome of what was called *iki* – chic. Not for her the gaudy padded kimono emblazoned with dragons embroidered in gold thread. The line of her kimono was simple, flowing and elegant and she always sacrificed comfort for style. It was the height of *iki* to go without stockings in the depths of winter, stepping out of the rickshaw into the snow with a tiny foot frozen inside its eye-catching black lacquered, high-soled clog. Or if she wore the traditional white split-toed socks, to choose a size too small so it would fit skin-tight and flatter the shape of her foot. *Iki* does not depend on physical beauty. It is everything that is daring and original, a quality that only increases with age as a woman tastes the bittersweet fruits of love and grows in confidence, wit and worldly knowledge. So it is no wonder that the experienced women of the water trade were more sought after than their young apprentices, and a geisha could not be said to have reached her prime until she was in her fifties or even her sixties. A refreshing and exciting thought for women of that age in the Western world.

Dressing with *iki* was a complicated business that required help from the *okasan*, the teahouse 'mother' and her maids. Nearest to her skin the geisha wore a traditional undergarment called a *koshimaki*, a length of fine silk simply wrapped around the waist. Next came a front-wrapping undershirt in fine cotton, then a silk under-robe and finally a kimono in delicate damask. Colours and patterns were carefully chosen to reflect subtle changes in the season and the mood of the wearer, following the formal language of the kimono that spoke so eloquently to the educated men who frequented the geishas' world. The kimono was secured with an *obi*, a broad belt of ornate brocade, wrapped around the geisha's waist to cover her from armpits to hips; the *okasan* drew it tight to the point of dizziness and tied it with a woven cord. After the geisha had dressed, her maids coiffed her hair with camellia nut oil and heated spatulas.

The kimono chastely flattened the geisha's breasts and wrapped high at the neck, but behind at the nape, it dipped, giving a tantalizing glimpse of the silk under-robe in a startling flash of pure colour, perhaps hot pink or scarlet. The delicate nape of the neck with its fine downy hairs holds a particular fascination for Japanese men. The geisha played upon this cleverly when she made up her face, taking the alabaster white foundation around the back of the neck, but leaving a lick of bare skin, reminiscent of both a serpent's tongue and the female private parts, to mesmerize the eyes of her admirers. She left a narrow border of bare skin around her hairline too, to serve as a reminder that behind the mask of illusion there was a real flesh–and–blood woman.

Finally, she applied kohl to her eyes and painted a narrow rosebud for a mouth. She took a booklet of powder papers from a fold in her obi and tore off a delicate sheet to powder her nose. The geisha knew that where magic is concerned, the appearance creates the reality.

Like nuns, geishas have always been a magnet for curiosity and speculation. A girl's life as a geisha often began when she was sold as a child to the geisha house, where she performed chores and ran errands until, around her fourteenth birthday, she was old enough to become an apprentice. The trainee geisha was called a *maiko*, and she was recognized by her shyness, her more demure hair-style and her long swinging sleeves – the sign of a virgin. Sometimes the *maiko* lost her virginity to a wealthy patron of the geisha house who paid the *okasan* a fabulous sum for the privilege of sleeping with her. Her initiation would take several nights, the man talking tenderly to her, showing her books of erotic art and massaging her thighs until she was eager to receive him. But sometimes a *maiko* graduated to geishahood while still a virgin. It was her choice. Most geishas refused to give themselves without love and passion.

The *maiko* often earned the money to pay for her training by working in the silk industry, feeding silkworms, unravelling their cocoons for spinning, or unfurling long bolts of freshly dyed silks and rinsing them in the river. She had to learn many skills, not least of which was how to sit and walk with elegance while wearing the restricting kimono, sliding one foot, pigeon-toed, just in front of the other, taking tiny steps with knees slightly bent. She learned to sing and dance and play the *shamisen*, an instrument like a lute with gold fittings, ivory pegs and a drum made from the skin of a virgin kitten – perfect and untouched by a tomcat's claws. She learned the intricate rules of the tea ceremony, and studied etiquette. An elaborate code of manners was essential in the geisha's twilight world of eroticism, for it set a tone of lightness and warmth, flirtation and gaiety in which men both knew their place and felt appreciated and admired for their good looks, brilliance and charm. The etiquette of greetings and formalities gave a structure to conversation that even the most tongue-tied of the geisha's admirers could fall back on, and created an atmosphere of glamour edged in discipline that is purely Japanese.

It was part of the geisha's mystique that though she was the most talented of hostesses, she never shared food with her clients. At a banquet she would pour the wine, deftly bone a fish or peel a grape, pampering utterly the man she was attending. Late at night, the party over, she returned home to the kitchen of the geisha house. There she sat and discussed the evening's adventures with her adopted sisters, as they ate leftover rice and drank jasmine tea, their feet tucked cosily under a table with a charcoal brazier burning beneath it.

The culture and traditions of India, China and Japan have been steeped in Tantra and the Tao of sex for thousands of years. Less well known is that in the Middle Ages these sexual teachings found their way into Europe, where they formed the foundation of the erotic religion known as Courtly Love. The high-born lovers who dedicated their lives to the transforming power of their passion developed the Tantric arts to suit their own culture, setting up a unique code of behaviour for reaching erotic and spiritual ecstasy.

Knowledge of Tantra had filtered through the East to Arabia, then crossed with the Moors to Spain. In the eleventh century Andalucia was captivated by the haunting strains of mystical Arab love songs. They idealized the purifying pain and suffering of earthly passion as a path to spiritual perfection. Composing their own love poetry and romantic ballads, Spanish minstrels called troubadours began travelling north into France, earning their keep by singing of longing, adoration, lust and loss. Their songs worshipped the elusive beloved as an erotic goddess, placing her on a pedestal of pure desire. The troubadours became the mainstream of medieval culture and their message inspired a flood of lyricism and song. This was the Tantric revolution of Courtly Love – the recognition that in sexual relations the woman holds the power. Among the upper classes at least, women were no longer the object of their lovers' pleasure but the instigators of the game.

The troubadours' bawdy songs and laments of unrequited love were music indeed to the ears of the nobility in whose castles and courts they performed. In an era of marriages arranged for political and economic reasons while the husband- and wife-to-be were still children, true adult passion was almost always adulterous. Courtly Love was incompatible with marriage, an institution designed to secure the male line of descent. In marriage, sex was a duty and a means to an end. Courtly Love was driven by eroticism and desire. When sex is no longer for procreation and love is free of obligation, the woman becomes the equal of the man. But when her marriage to another makes her inaccessible, she becomes his goddess. The cult of the unattainable Lady ran parallel to the cult of the Virgin Mary, with which it had striking similarities. In both cases the exaltation of desire motivated the lover and filled him with power.

It is a mistake to suppose that the Lady of medieval romance was a wan and passive creature. In fact Courtly Love was the one arena of life in the Middle Ages in which the female sex not only enjoyed rights and dues, but reigned supreme. Within marriage a woman had to submit to her husband, but in Courtly Love it was she who made the choice and granted the favours. In pursuit of her regard, her admirer had to attune his desires to hers at every stage of the courtship.

Noblewomen also used their natural expertise in psychology to become judges in matters of love.

The Romantic movement had its heart at Poitiers, at the brilliant court of Queen Eleanor of Aquitaine. The Queen and her daughter Countess Marie of Troyes set up and presided over secret courts of love, in which they and their ladies sat in judgment on cases of romantic intrigue, jealousy and betrayal. These courts were the only place where adulterous liaisons were recognized as having any social status. Cases were brought before the courts of love by a third party, a confidant of the plaintiff, who was forbidden to reveal the names of the parties concerned, at least until a judgment had been reached. The Queen and her jury examined the evidence, then made their deliberations according to the code of Courtly Love, which they devised and which was later written down by Andreas Capellanus. They offered sympathetic counselling to wronged lovers and punished offenders by banishing them from high society.

The risks of entering an adulterous relationship were high, especially for women who feared the wrath of their husbands. Queen Eleanor's code of Courtly Love contained practical advice to guard against discovery. She urged lovers never to sign secret letters and to select a trusted friend or servant to be a messenger, go–between and confidant. A certain amount of voyeurism was attached to this role; it gave rise to the expression 'to hold a candle for someone', which meant to help with a love affair, and to the title of 'secretary', originally the keeper of secrets. There was always a danger of the secretary becoming too intimately involved, but since adulterous love thrives on fear and jealousy, the threat of betrayal added to the piquancy of the affair. However, the Queen cautioned against allowing more than one person to hold the candle, or the whole edifice of secrecy would quickly disintegrate.

Courtly lovers trod a delicate path between truth and falsehood. They were fired by the purity of their love, yet their assignations were built on lies and deceit. The only solution was to live parallel lives. The lovers were to guard the honour of those they deceived by allowing no hint or rumour of the affair to reach their ears, and by behaving towards them with the utmost deference and respect. But between themselves in their intimate paradise there were to be no secrets, lies or falsehoods. The paradox of adulterous love and of paradise itself is its isolation from reality, for it cannot be held onto or brought into the everyday world, and flourishes only in the elusive realm of sensuality and dreams. Thus the dawn song – the most popular ballad of the troubadours – became the anthem and the symbol of the Romantic movement. Crystallized within it was all the lovers' ecstasy, only heightened by the agony of parting at daybreak. They met for the duration of a brief embrace, but their embrace lasted for all eternity.

From the poets and troubadours who gathered at their court, Queen Eleanor and Marie of Troyes commissioned epic romances that expressed the essence of Courtly Love. These great works of humanity and imagination centred on the passion of a knight for his Lady. To prove himself worthy of her notice, he excelled as a poet and storyteller or performed feats of skill and daring, and heroic deeds in battle. But because an easy conquest robs love of its charm, the Lady scorned him with cruel words; she knew that keeping him balanced between hope and fear would spur him on to even greater achievements. And her suitor could refuse his beloved nothing, because it lay in her power to give him all.

With her image as his guide and inspiration, the knight vowed to surpass and transcend himself in the name of love. So he embarked on the always perilous journey of self-discovery. On the way through this most treacherous of landscapes he fought dragons and monsters, which were the manifestations of his own weaknesses and internal demons. He slew a giant wielding a formidable phallic club. This towering figure represented the authority of his father, and all the taboos that blocked the fulfilment of his dreams. He set sail on water, the feminine element, and was immediately blown every which way, lost at sea in a sea of love. He entered a parched wasteland, where love was denied him and he suffered untold miseries of thirst. Finally, after surviving many trials and tribulations, he passed through a dark forest and found himself in an enchanted garden. Here in this secret paradise his Lady waited.

The separations and tests that they had endured served only to refine and strengthen their passion, and the lovers came together charged with erotic longing. The poet drew a veil of secrecy across the ecstasy of their meeting. But the name of the quintessential hero of medieval romance was Tristan, which gave the reader the clue that the couple practised the *Tantric* arts of love.

The poet – Chrétien de Troyes – revealed that Tristan and his beloved slept with his sword between them. He practised the art of withholding. Coitus was forbidden in the strict framework of the lovers' code. This was not just to avoid the risk of pregnancy revealing their secret, but because intercourse was the essence of marriage, with all its connotations of invasion, conquest and possession. In Courtly Love it was vital that the woman was not conquered but remained replete in all her mysteries.

In courtship the knight had devoted himself to fulfilling his Lady's every desire, and now he held back while he satisfied her body and soul with a thousand caresses. Though the courtly lovers did not practise penetrative sex, they indulged rapturously in the countless other delights of erotic love-play. The songs of the troubadours celebrated the pleasures of 'lechery', from the French for 'to lick', and Tristan was said to play the harp with consummate skill, a hint of the magic in his sensitive fingers. The interplay of adoration and eroticism, the urging on and the holding back, were a perfect expression of Tantric sexuality. In Courtly Love as in Tantra, man and woman were destined to continually satisfy and complete each other. The knight's Tantric self–control meant that the lovers could make love all night long, each experiencing many peaks of ecstasy, until dawn broke and the Lady finally vanquished him, his semen as bright and final as the light that streaked the sky.

Just as the courtly lovers of the Age of Romance adapted the sexual practices of Tantra and the Tao to suit their own culture, so there is a way of bring– ing the lost erotic wisdom of the East into the lives of modern men and women. And that way is called the path to the Seventh Heaven.

The
Conversation

The secret is to realize that the sacred lies in the ordinary. It is the way you value your life that counts. The richness of your experience lies in your reactions and not in the parade that passes before your eyes.

ADAM LOOKED UP FROM THE parchment scroll at Eve, who lay on the bed beside him, cupping her chin in her hands. Deciphering the delicate handwriting in faded ink seemed to have affected his eyes. He felt as if he had dozed off, but now he was suddenly alert, awake to a gathering energy, an air of expectation in the room. Eve appeared to sense it too, for she turned her head; his spine tingled as he followed her gaze. In the dim light at the foot of the bed, colours were stirring, a shiver of electricity caught at iridescent purples and greens. And gradually as they watched, the ethereal figures of three women evolved before them as if painted in light.

One of them moved forward. 'I am Koriko', said the apparition, bowing deeply, 'a geisha of the Floating World. We three are the authors of the parchment that you hold in your hands.'

'My name is Marguerite', said the second figure. 'In my earthly life I was a lady-in-waiting to Queen Eleanor of Aquitaine. By reading our words you have called us from our rest. We are here to impart to you the secrets of our erotic traditions and to bring you sexual wisdom from across the ancient world.'

'I am Padmini', said the third, amid a brilliance of jewels, 'a courtesan of classical India, a rare companion to diplomats and princes of the realm. We are your guides on a journey of erotic adventure, which is called the pathway to the Seventh Heaven.'

Adam and Eve exchanged glances. 'A journey?' said Adam.

'A journey that will deepen your desire, strengthen your sexual energy and immeasurably increase ecstasy and fulfilment', promised Koriko. 'On your journey you will pass through seven gate–ways, which you will read about in our seven scrolls. At each gateway, we will meet you and instruct you. Today we meet at the first step on your journey, which is called The Gateway to Heaven'.

'Are you going to teach us Tantric sex positions?' asked Eve doubtfully.

Padmini smiled. 'Certainly you will learn secrets from Tantra and the Tao that are of real value in modern life, but we shall leave yogic sex for the pleasure of the gods and the yogis. In fact, for the duration of your journey, we shall forsake sex completely ...'

'An erotic journey without sex?'

Koriko giggled at Adam's expression. 'You see, for most couples, coitus signifies the beginning of the end of the erotic encounter. And it brings with it the potential for so many complex problems and anxieties. On your journey to the Seventh Heaven you will leave these anxieties behind as you discover how to deepen your erotic awareness and intensify your responses to each other.'

'The main problem that couples face,' explained Marguerite, 'is that sex is over relatively rapidly for a man, while for a woman it is a continuum that can last for hours. And dissatisfaction that starts in the bedroom has a habit of colouring the rest of life. The pathway to the Seventh Heaven frees sex from objectives and goals, thereby taking away the pressure to perform.

'On your journey, you will explore the warmth and nourishment that derive from intimate language and behaviour, and the many different ways of caressing with the whole body, hands and mouths. Besides,' she smiled, 'learning restraint is erotic in itself. And so that you can prolong your intimacy still further, we will teach Adam the ancient sexual arts of delaying ejaculation.'

'Both of you will gain in confidence from practising stress-free sexuality,' said Koriko. 'It means that you will be able to enjoy each other at any time and for any length of time, without precautions or side–effects, and with total erotic bliss.'

'And after you have passed through the final gateway of your journey and come together again as bride and groom,' said Padmini, 'your passion and excitement in sex will be as fresh and intense as when you first met, but deeper and longer–lasting.'

'I want to make this journey,' said Adam, 'but will it be worth the effort? Is the business of ejaculation control really something I could work at and achieve?'

'Effort is a purely Western concept,' said Koriko. 'Let me tell you a story to show what I mean. It's the story of a princess shut up in a tall tower with no door, and a prince who fell in love with her. He couldn't climb the tower, as its walls were smooth as glass. He couldn't beat them down as they were strong as iron. He couldn't reach her with a ladder because there were no ladders long enough. So he took a silken thread and tied one end of it to a snail, which climbed very slowly up to the waiting princess. She untied the thread and began to pull it up. The prince tied a length of string to the thread. When she pulled up the string, he tied a length of rope to the end of it. She hauled up the rope, secured it in the tower, and he climbed up to her.

'So now you see the gentleness and subtlety with which great things are naturally and comfortably achieved. The Western way would be to batter frantically at the door or to hurl a heavy rope up into the air hoping the princess could catch it. These attempts would involve effort and frustration, disappointment and pain. The Eastern way is all about relaxing and conserving energy.

'Through your study of the seven scrolls you will learn to open your mind to many new sensations. Gradually, as you relax into a deeper knowledge of your sexuality, you will discover how to conserve the energy of ejaculation and redirect it to prolong your lovemaking. The path to the Seventh Heaven is so full of erotic delight that you will be unaware of learning anything at all until you discover how you have changed!'

'Why is it called the Seventh Heaven?' asked Eve. 'What's so special about the number seven?'

'There are seven days in each of the four phases of the moon,' said Padmini, 'so the number seven belongs to the eternal goddess, to sexuality and to the cycle of fertility, all of which are ruled by the moon.'

'The ancients said that when the soul ascended into paradise, it climbed a ladder of seven rungs, and passed through seven heavens, the spheres of the planets that still rule our lives in the seven days of the week,' said Marguerite. 'And in the ancient world when sex and religion were one, the word *climax* actually meant "ladder to heaven" – climbing the seven-runged ladder to erotic bliss and mystic enlightenment. In Tantra and Taoism the rungs of the heavenly ladder were found in the worshipper's own spiritual body. They are the seven chakras, the energy centres of the spine.'

'The mystic ascent of the seven-runged ladder is still celebrated today in the Hindu marriage ceremony,' said Padmini. 'The priest ties the hem of the bride's sari to the groom's scarf to bind them in wedlock and together they walk seven times around the sacred fire as the groom chants the marriage mantra. They take seven steps: the first for food, the second for strength, the third for prosperity, the fourth for happiness, the fifth for children, the sixth for pleasure and the seventh for love and companionship.'

'Is it necessary to be religious to climb the ladder to the Seventh Heaven?' asked Adam.

'Not in the way you think,' said Padmini. 'Though Tantra is a spiritual path, it doesn't call on its followers to renounce pleasure and mortify the flesh, which is why it is so scandalous to orthodox religions. On the contrary, its aim is to raise erotic pleasure to the peak of human experience in a blaze of spiritual energy. In the West, you expect the intensity of sexual experience to wane after a few years. The path to the Seventh Heaven will show you how to regain this transcendent happiness so that your whole lives are full of positive energy.

'Awareness is the key, opening the mind to love, and discovering greater levels of eroticism and desire. Giving up intercourse for the duration of the seven steps will allow you to slow down and immerse yourselves in sensuality. To make love with honour and tenderness is the spiritual path to the Seventh Heaven, and to revel in sexual excitement without the tension of having to prove yourself or reach any goals. This is the meditative approach that will generate renewed passion.'

'Do we have to learn meditation?' asked Eve.

'It is not necessary,' said Marguerite. 'However, meditation is good for dissolving many of the obstacles that block the way to sexual happiness. I'm thinking of stress, loss of humour, argu-mentative behaviour and irritability, indecision and forgetfulness, the inability to listen or relax, and the torture of having problems niggling constantly round and round in your head.

'Meditation also helps on the path to the Seventh Heaven by increasing sensual and spiritual awareness. Simply by sitting still in a comfortable cross-legged position, with spine erect, shoulders dropped, eyes closed and your hands resting on your thighs, whilst concentrating only on the gentle ebb and flow of your breath, you can become aware of the most minute sensations. If you practise this – doing absolutely nothing! – for a few minutes every day, you will soon start to connect with your spiritual body. You may feel the skin tingle or the scalp crawl. A glow of heat sometimes builds up inside the chest, or coloured lights start to scribble and flash in front of your closed eyes. Perhaps there will be sensations like fine electrical cobwebs brushing against your skin, or a fuzzy numbness.'

'This electrical energy that Marguerite is describing is the life force we call *qi* or *chi*,' said Koriko. 'You will be familiar with it already in some of the mysterious emotional responses of the body, such as butterflies in the stomach, a heavy heart, a lump in the throat, or a tingling sensation in the spine and scalp. And, of course, in the ecstasy of orgasm, the body's most concentrated expression of energy.'

'All these sensations take place along the spine at the chakras', said Padmini. 'The orgasm takes place at the root chakra, the butterflies of nervousness in the solar plexus, emotional heaviness or lightness in the heart chakra, sadness at the throat chakra, and the thrill of fear or excitement runs up the whole spine, joining all the chakras together.'

'Meditation is just one of the ways of connecting with *chi*', said Koriko. 'If you want to find out more about how to use this natural universal power to boost your sexual energy and minimize stress and tension, I would encourage you to take up an Eastern form of exercise, whether it be martial arts, *t'ai chi*, *chi gung* or yoga. All of these disciplines will help you cultivate real internal strength – physical, emotional, mental, spiritual and sexual.'

'Is it a failure to need instruction in the art of love?' wondered Eve.

'By no means!' said Marguerite. 'Making love may be a simple act between two people, but it is complicated in every way by society. By censure and gossip, by worries about what is normal and acceptable, by idealization, obsession and anxiety. Although sex is a natural activity, it's not as natural as breathing. It develops with practice, like any other art, and the detail of making love unfolds uniquely to each new pair of lovers. Yet in time, pleasure tends to grow stale. And this is why the ancients developed the knowledge that we are here to give you, and why, since written records began, lovers have consulted guides to help them.'

'What is the secret of not getting stale?' asked Adam. 'Is it to do with novelty and variety?'

'Novelty and variety have their value,' said Koriko, 'but in time, they too become stale, and the constant search for new diversions grows wearing. The secret is to realize that the sacred lies in the ordinary. It is the way you value your life that counts. The richness of your experience lies in your reactions and not in the parade that passes before your eyes.'

'Honour yourself,' said Marguerite. 'Treat yourself as you would want to be treated. Yes, you look surprised, but learning to love yourself will make you more lovable. So, we will give you some very down-to-earth advice. Make sure you eat well, whether you are together or apart. Love your body. Pamper yourself; take care with your appearance. Find clothes that suit you, and create your own individual style. Choose underwear and nightwear with as much care as the rest of your wardrobe. Look after your skin and hair. Pay attention to your hands. Be happy, be gorgeous, cultivate and take delight in your inner self.'

'Don't worry about your age,' said Koriko. 'Remember a geisha doesn't start to reach her prime until her fifties!'

'Enjoy physical pleasures,' said Padmini. 'Exercise,

bathing, the eroticism of eating, of preparing and sharing food. Go dancing, or dance together at home. Lose yourselves in the power of dance; let it raise your spirits to the point of ecstasy.'

'Indulge in small acts of kindness,' said Marguerite. 'Draw a blind to keep the sun out of your lover's eyes, fetch a cushion or a drink. Make a surprise out of a delicious and imaginatively pre- pared snack. Give a small but perfectly chosen gift. Offer a neck massage, or play some music to help your lover unwind.'

'Try to get rid of narrow perceptions of gender,' said Koriko. 'Romance is not just for women, and nor are chores. It's good for men to explore their feminine qualities and women their masculine side. It improves the balance between the male and the female in the relationship as well as within oneself.'

'And talking of romance,' said Padmini, 'the grand romantic gesture is not always as appropriate as simple kindness and consideration. Tune in to your lover and discover where you can offer practical help. Then just do it without fuss. Remember the sacred lies in the ordinary.'

'Talk together,' said Marguerite. 'Voice your problems instead of brooding. Ask questions to delve deeper and relieve tension when your partner is feeling low. Don't forget to say "I love you". Pay attention and notice everything. Make eye contact. Be fully in the present and engage.'

'Pay compliments,' said Padmini. 'Appreciate your lover's wit and intelligence, kindness, sensuality and charm. Admire their appearance and achievements. Avoid the temptation to criticize or compete. Remember moments of intimacy together.'

'Make your bedroom a private place,' said Koriko, 'a refuge from the outside word where no distractions come between you. Make it calm, with clear uncluttered lines that your eyes can rest on without agitation. Enjoy the comfort of fresh, natural fabrics. Pay attention to lighting. Soft lamplight throws flattering shadows. In *feng shui*, the far right–hand corner of the room opposite the door is the relationship corner. What you have in that corner may tell you something interesting. Perhaps you could place some flowers there or something beautiful that is precious to you.'

'Endearments spoken or whispered from the heart have a tremendous seductive power,' said Padmini. 'And pillow talk is much easier if you have a vocabulary you are both comfortable with. Honour your sexual parts by giving them names. The English names are not erotic – they are either too clinical or too crass. In Sanskrit, the world's earliest language, the vulva was called the *yoni*, which means "sacred place", and the penis was the *lingam*, the "wand of light" or the *vajra*, the "tool of consciousness". Using your own erotic vocabulary is a great aphrodisiac and it will enable you to ask for what you want in bed. Ask what your lover wants too, and enjoy the game of giving detailed instructions, as if it was all completely new to you.'

'In bed you can use all your senses in appreciating how your beloved looks, smells, feels, tastes and sounds,' said Marguerite. 'I adored the sound of kisses, I loved to hear my beloved sighing or groaning with desire. Feast your eyes on each other. The eyes, as everyone knows, are the window of the soul.'

'Keep the connection between you when lovemaking is over,' said Koriko. 'The slow, erotic build-up and the gentle, affectionate letting-down are truly essential arts of romance.'

The light in the room seemed to falter. The apparitions at the foot of the bed started to fade.

'And now,' said Padmini, 'forget everything we have told you. For in the words of the *Kamasutra*, "When the wheel of ecstasy is in full motion, there is no textbook at all, and no order."'

With that the three courtesans were gone. Eve took Adam's hand and kissed it. Their erotic journey had begun . . .

SCROLL 2

A Drift of Petals

❦

The Courtesans' Parchment

All Eastern philosophies
recognize and honour the stillness
that lies at the heart of action.
Rest and a sense of timelessness
are part of the Eastern way
of life.

T OUCH IS THE MOST HUMAN AND THE MOST basic of all the senses. In the Eastern traditions, ritual touching in the form of massage has been part of daily life for thousands of years. Indian infants are gently massaged every day from birth with a dough ball dipped into warm almond oil. After the age of six, children share massage with family members, learning how to touch and be touched in a healing and comforting way. Massage has long played a vital role in Japanese life, and is often practised in the relaxed atmosphere of the *sento*, the public baths, on relatives, friends and strangers. The Japanese have a word for the way touch bonds and grounds people, making them equal: *sukinshippu* – 'skinship'.

Many types of massage practised in the East can be given without undressing or much preparation. In China and Japan *tui-na* and *anma*, the forerunners of modern shiatsu, are performed on family members by pressing with the palms and thumbs along pathways called meridians to harmonize the life energy that flows through the body. Knowledge of the many benefits of these practices to body, mind and spirit is passed down from one generation to the next. Indian head massage was originally developed by women as a beauty therapy they could share. They rubbed aromatic oils into each other's scalps to keep their hair strong and lustrous. Barbers began to offer the same service to their male clients. The firm gentle rhythm of shampooing resolves blockages, melts troubles and opens up pathways of communication and understanding. The practitioners of *champi*, as it was known, listened to people's problems as they teased them out of their hair. Perhaps if people in the

Western world did this for each other on a regular basis their lives would be the happier.

The Indian medical system of ayurveda, which means 'the science of life', prescribes many wonderful specialist massages. These include clay baths, hot herbal poultices, and *dhara*, a treatment in which a warm healing oil is poured in a stream onto the receiver's forehead and rubbed into the hair and scalp to diminish the effects of ageing. In this culture, particular care has always been lavished on bride and groom before their wedding. Indian brides are traditionally readied for the marriage bed by forty days of massage and beauty treatments that leave their limbs pliant and supple and their skin soft and lustrous, culminating in the *ubtan* massage for fertility and long-lasting health on the eve of the wedding.

In their separate houses the bride and groom are covered in a festive paste made of ground nuts and gram flour mixed with oil and spices, especially turmeric, which is known to stimulate the production of hormones as well as to guard against disease. The oil lubricates the skin and the paste draws out the heat and any impurities with it as it dries. As the paste is rubbed off with small circling movements of the fingers, the tissues are stimulated, the circulation is enhanced and fresh energy is drawn to the surface of the skin. The massage is followed by a sun bath and a dip in cool water spiked with lemon juice. The luxurious treatment rejuvenates the body and stills the mind in preparation for the momentous day ahead.

All Eastern philosophies recognize and honour the stillness that lies at the heart of action. Rest and a sense of timelessness are part of the Eastern way of life. In the West time is a commodity, a rare and highly priced luxury, and life is lived under a press-ing sense of urgency. Not enough time means constant low-level stress. Stress leads to a negative attitude – *I can't cope* – which results in insomnia and fatigue. The joints tense and natural radiance is lost. Stimulants are used so that more activity can be crammed into less time. The result is a lowering of immunity and faster ageing, not to mention earlier death.

Stress is the enemy of erotic love because it blocks the mind, exhausts the will and overloads the body with toxins, making it tense and jumpy. Stress and tension are the major ills of modern society and need addressing every day. In the East massage has long been practised to release into vitality and health the energy that is harmfully held in tension. The benefits of massage are without number. It improves the texture and tone of the skin. Stiff muscles relax, painful areas are soothed, toxins excreted. It enhances the circulation of nutrients and oxygen, improving the digestion and increasing immunity. It induces calm and relax-ation, balance and harmony. It triggers the release of hormones that raise sexual responsiveness. And where words cannot quell irrational anxieties, the hand of comfort can often heal insecurity and instil confidence.

The mystery of knowing another human being through the art of touch lies in putting the awareness into the hands, to make them super-sensitive to the skin, and opening the mind to the flesh, muscle, blood, nerves, bone, and above all the emotions of the other. But it has long been understood in the East that touching does not just take place on a physical level. It is also the interplay of two energetic fields. The intention we put into our hands is just as important as their ability to listen. In Eastern medicine, the therapist's hands are used on the body with the intention to resolve and balance the energetic disturbances detected there. The combination of sensitivity to touch and projection of good intentions into the body of another person need not be restricted to healers. It is something that anyone can develop with practice through massage. Touch makes feelings a reality.

In the modern Western world there are countless taboos against the instinctive human language of touch. The formalized rituals of massage give permission to touch someone within established and well–defined boundaries. They also give licence to explore to the limit of those boundaries and experiment with new sensations. Learning how to massage opens up the art of touch in an exciting way that can be brought into everyday life to maintain health, resolve stress, and keep close to the beloved, so that erotic caressing always feels natural and free.

The
Conversation

Illusion sets the imagination free,

its tendrils uncurl as all the senses

come to life in its luxuriant

warmth.

*W*HEN ADAM AND EVE LOOKED UP after reading the second scroll of the courtesans' parchment, they found themselves in a dimly lit room in old Japan. They were not alone.

'In Japan we love the mystery of darkness,' said Koriko. 'Not for us the glare of sunlight or the harsh brilliance of an electric lamp. We prefer the soft living glow of candles, their flames trembling with the faintest draught, flooding the moving contours of the body with drifting shadows, like a caress. As your eyes relax into the darkness of this room, they will open to many subtle layers of darkness, the rich darkness seen only by candlelight.

'At the furthest reaches of your vision – in the corners of the room and the heavy folds of the curtain – the deep unfathomable velvet blackness soaks away your thoughts and cares, stilling the eyes and the mind with its infinite profundity. Through the muted darkness of this screen you observe the pale glimmer of tea lights in another part of the house. The dim space outside the candle glow is alive with infinitesimal motes of blackness, falling; open your eyes wider and you sense in them a mesmerizing shower of dark iridescent colour.

'In Japan we know how to use the darkness as a spell; we know how to fill it with secrets. See how the gold leaf shimmers in the flickering flame, rest your eyes on the dull lustre of this bowl as I turn it in the light. Observe the faint glint of the ornaments in the blackness of my hair, the way my white-painted face floats towards you on the darkness like a flower kissed by moonshine: this is the enchant-ment of the dark. If you were to turn on an electric light, its glare would chase the secrets from their shadows; the gold leaf, the lustre, the lacquer, the brilliant hues of my kimono would leap forward and wound your eyes with their garishness. The delicate pallor of my face would seem lifeless and hard. In the dark we create illusion. Illusion sets the imagination free, its tendrils uncurl as all the senses come to life in its luxuriant warmth. And as we float in the sensuous realm of the imagination, anchored in the present yet drifting, we pass through the second gateway on your erotic journey, in which we explore the delights of the art of touch in all its subtle nuances.'

'The caress begins in the imagination,' said Padmini. 'The imagination takes hints from glimmers in the darkness and then feasts in hedonistic ecstasy on what the eye cannot see. In your modern world, where naked flesh is on display everywhere, the imagination is quickly sated, soon jaded.'

'Let your bedroom be a room full of shadows,'

said Marguerite, 'shadows that fall between you like a veil, caressing the curves and hollows of your bodies, inviting the hand to follow. The veil of mystery is the most tempting invitation.'

Padmini turned to Eve. 'Now we approach the second gateway on your path to the Seventh Heaven, the art of touch. Arouse your lover's desire to touch you by learning the art of suggestion in your dress. Offer his eyes a subtle clue as to what lies beneath, but no more. Allow him to believe that only he can read its erotic message. See how Koriko's kimono wraps demurely at the throat? Her dark sparkling eyes command full attention. But see how the fabric dips at the nape, revealing that most tender and vulnerable part of the female anatomy that Japanese men so love to kiss. Only as she turns to go is the promise glimpsed, leaving her wistful lover to sigh *ahh . . . but now it is too late!* This is part of Koriko's erotic mystique.

'Now consider my own mode of dress. You see how the sari bodice is cut to the exact shape of my breasts, but then the voluptuous tailoring all but disappears from the gaze beneath a veil of silk. My navel, which in many cultures as well as my own represents the clitoris, is pierced with a jewel; its sparkle of fire and the smooth contours of my belly are just visible to the hungry eye that penetrates the filmy gauze of my wrap. Perhaps it has never occurred to you that the exquisite swirling robes and loose trousers that form traditional dress in the East, covering us from head to toe, are yet perfectly designed for accessibility? The girls from my village could make love quite openly in the fields without taking anything off. And so it was that my prince and I could enjoy each other fully clothed in a pavilion in the palace garden, as our attentive servants stood close by, looking on. No matter how hard they stared, they could not see all. The flagrant secrecy of it set us on fire. Think of these things, both of you, when you choose how to dress for love.'

'The women of northern Europe knew nothing of

these seductive tricks until the Middle Ages,' confided Marguerite. 'We used to wear voluminous tunics of coarse cloth similar to men's, and in bed both sexes wore a *chemise cagoule*, a long nightshirt with a hole in the front to accommodate marital duty. But when the Crusaders returned from the East they brought exciting news of women showing off their figures with a low-cut bodice that swooped beneath the bust and fastened at the front with tight lacing right down to the hips. Underneath it was a fine chemise that barely concealed the breasts before falling softly to the ankles.

'From these most enticingly dressed women our knights had learned the secrets of Tantric love. They came home inspired, and showered us with gifts of jewels and exotic perfumes, aphrodisiac spices, rich cloths from Phrygia, Damascus and Constantinople, costly Saracen silks and brocades. We sewed the sensuous fabrics as we listened enthralled to tales of caresses erotic beyond our dreams. For the first time we wore dresses that both restricted and revealed our bodies. The contrast, you see, between the offering and the denial is what excites men's desire. Use this knowledge, Eve, in the way you dress during the day. Let your sexuality speak through your clothes. It will transform the way you feel about yourself and make men long to touch you, as I can vouch. The new fashion awakened all our senses and spread like fire across Europe; the ideals of Courtly Love sprang from our whispered conversations.'

'In the East we have a long and sacred tradition of caring lovingly for our own bodies,' said Padmini. Her bangles glittered in the candlelight as she turned a smooth bare arm for their admiration. The arm seemed to move of its own accord with sinuous, snakelike grace. 'A supple body and a lively mind are the best preparations for learning the arts of love,' she said. 'My daily yoga and deep breathing exercises flush my mind and body with vitality. We care for our skin – men as well as women – with healing oils and rejuvenating massage treatments that make it glow and tingle with health. Learn to look after and appreciate your skin, this precious organ of touch.'

'Turn your daily bath into a heavenly delight,' said Koriko. 'There are five ingredients that transform the "raven's bath", as we call it in Japan – no more than a brief splash in a puddle – into a sensual ritual that calms and clears the mind as much as it refreshes the body, making it the perfect prelude for love. These ingredients are to exfoliate, stimulate, relax, refresh and moisturize.

'Friction exfoliates the skin, sloughing off dead cells and leaving it vibrant and fresh. Pay particular attention to the feet, which are often a problem with men.' She cast a glance at Adam. 'Rub the heels and the sides of the feet gently with a pumice stone. Rub your back, shins and elbows with a sea–grass mitten.'

'Another way to exfoliate is to use a body brush before you bathe,' said Marguerite. 'Always brush towards the heart. This has the effect of stimulating the circulation, which in turn increases sensitivity to touch, something that doesn't happen with a wet facecloth.'

'The circulation and the skin are also stimulated by a change of temperature, a feature of the bathing routine in many cultures,' said Padmini. 'In the Turkish *hammam* a steam bath is followed by a cool dip. The public baths of Rome were heated to four different temperatures. The second and third baths were each hotter than the one before and the final bath provided a refreshing cold contrast. Heat dilates the blood vessels and cold contracts them, and the two actions together get the blood moving vibrantly round the body and the skin tingling with health.'

'The relaxing soak is probably what you most look forward to in a bath,' said Koriko, 'but have you ever considered the wisdom of soaking in dirty water, which is exactly what most people do?' And she told them how a Japanese bather soaps up and rinses off with a shower hose while sitting on a small stool before getting into the tub to soak. Thus the bathwater is kept perfectly clean and fragrant, and washing is a separate activity to the meditative luxury of relaxing. The ritual ends with a cool shower, a fresh kimono and a soothing cup of jasmine tea. Koriko's dark eyes sparkled in the dimly lit room as she described the delights of wallowing in a wooden tub gently heated from below by a wood stove. As she soaked, she would contemplate the moonlit river beneath her window and listen to the fragile music of wind chimes. Sometimes insect vendors came up from the country, selling crickets in cages so that city-dwellers like herself could enjoy cricket-listening ceremonies in the bath.

'How lovely!' said Eve. She was full of enthusiasm for a candlelit bath with wind chimes, and a com-bination of vigorous scrubbing under the shower followed by a long hot soak in fresh water, and a final cool rinse.

'In my tradition both men and women moisturize

the skin after bathing', said Padmini, 'to leave it smooth and supple with a delicate sheen, so that limbs glide sensuously against each other and bodies slip and slide in the caress. We use pure essential oils to scent the bath, to give healing and aphrodisiac power to a massage, and to moisturize. Perhaps you prefer a body lotion, but try just a light dab of perfumed oil at the base of the throat, on the pulse point inside the wrist, behind the knee, in the tender crease of the groin, or beneath the ear – it can be extremely erotic for both sexes. The Tantrics anointed their bodies before making love to awaken the senses and intensify emotional experience. They dabbed oil of sandalwood on the man's forehead, chest, underarms, navel and groin. His partner was anointed with jasmine on her wrists, patchouli at her neck, amber over her breasts, musk in her groin and saffron on her feet.'

'How does perfume work as an aphrodisiac?' Adam wanted to know.

'Pure perfume is distilled from flow

organs of plants,' said Padmini, 'and from precious resins secreted by trees and shrubs, such as myrrh, frankincense and styrax. These oils and resins contain substances very like the human hormones that awaken our desires when we detect them in the sweat and on the breath of our lovers. This is why perfumes and incense have such a potent effect on the human emotions – they overwhelm us with erotic messages and induce a swoon of ecstasy. When lovers caress, the scents of their breath and fresh beads of sweat begin to mingle with perfumes heated by their passion. The ancients believed that they could directly experience the divine by breathing in incense and perfumes. In Tantra, the religion of sex, sexual and religious ecstasy are one and the same.

'The seven chakras, the energy centres on the spine through which the spirit of ecstasy rises to bliss and enlightenment, are each associated with a particular scent. Musk for the root, then myrrh for the sacral chakra, amber for the solar plexus, rose for the heart, frankincense for the throat, jasmine for the third eye, and lotus for the crown. In the East we have recognized the chakras as whirling vortices of primal sexual energy for thousands of years, and within the last hundred years your Western scientists have discovered that they mirror almost exactly the position of the endocrine glands, which produce the hormones that give us our scents.'

'The nose is certainly the body's most underrated sex organ,' agreed Koriko. 'It detects hormones in perfume, on our breath and in our sweat, and it also reacts strongly to sexual excitement. Orgasm some-times causes a fit of sneezing and occasionally even a nosebleed. This is because it triggers a rapid dilation of the veins inside the nose, which makes the temperature there rise by nearly two degrees. The noses of people who are hypersensitive to smells sometimes feel blocked after sex. The ancient Chinese knew of this phenomenon and advised wrapping up well after orgasm to avoid catching a cold. And Roman physicians recommended giving up sex at the first sign of a cold or catarrh, as orgasm would only make it worse.' She lowered her voice. 'The Romans were well aware of the role played by smell in uncontrollable attractions – they punished adulterers by cutting off their noses!'

'The secret of the erotic caress is very simple,' said Marguerite. 'It lies in being fully aware physically and emotionally in the moment of contact. This is the single most important skill a lover needs to develop, far more valuable than any technique. However, it does take practice if you are to master it. It takes attention, concentration and relaxation. In the enveloping shadows of this room, as the candle flickers and the motes of darkness fall, let your shoulders sink, your arms, hands and fingers lengthen and relax. Half–close your eyes. Put all your awareness into your palms and fingertips ... perhaps you already feel some tingling there. As long as the awareness is in your hands, they are ready to give and to receive.'

'And now we discuss the art of massage,' said Padmini. 'The aim is not for you to become skilled masseurs, but to explore and enjoy each other's bodies with many different types of touch.'

'Massage means giving from the heart,' said Marguerite. 'Once you have learned the principles and the basic strokes, it's easy and your techniques and your routine will develop with practice. But don't save massage for special occasions – it's something you can share every day. You can give a head, neck and back massage in a few minutes with your partner sitting in a chair. You can massage the feet or hands as you sit and talk, and give a whole-body massage once or twice a week. You will soon notice an improvement in your well-being, the quality of your touch and your sexual vitality.'

'In my tradition, it is often blind people who become professional masseurs of the face and head,' said Padmini. 'Try it with your eyes half closed to develop your sensitivity. Hold the head still in both your hands before you begin. Circling and dragging strokes with the pads of the fingers feel gentle and comforting. Move both sets of fingers in time. Then try tapping and drumming the head with spread fingers, dropping the fingertips onto the scalp like rain.

'Your word *shampoo* comes from the Hindi word for massage, *champi*. Pull at the scalp and the roots of the hair with the fingertips, then shampoo with individually circling fingers all over the scalp. Gently ease the fingers through the strands of hair, working from the hairline at the back, supporting the forehead with the heel of the other hand. Vigorous movements stimulate and increase alert‑ness. Soft, slow, rhythmic movements release many tensions.'

'Just as the mind leads the hand, so your intention is transmitted by your touch', said Koriko. 'So let your thoughts dwell on relaxing, releasing and healing, and put your mind into your hands as you explore your partner's body with care and attention. Let the ease and well–being of your lover fill your mind, excluding all other thoughts.'

'Where is the best place to give a massage?' asked Eve.

'On a firm bed or, better still, on a quilt or futon on the floor,' said Koriko. 'Working on the floor in a kneeling position helps with grounding and calming, so important if you're both suffering from stress. In Japan we *live* on the floor for this very reason – we sit, sleep, eat, massage and make love at ground level.'

'Make your room warm and private,' said Marguerite. 'Clear away clutter – it jars on the eye and on the mind. Dim the light; burn a stick of incense or some aromatic oil. Spread out a fresh sheet to lie on. Have massage oil nearby and a light blanket to cover those parts of the body you are not working on, or a hot towel. The warmth may incubate desire.'

'How can we get the most out of being massaged?' asked Adam.

'To receive a massage, still your mind and focus on the sensations of being inside your body,' said Padmini. 'Close your eyes and relax. Imagine your body is made of feathers, then of water, then of billions of grains of sand. As it gets heavier and heavier, feel the tension draining out of your neck, shoulders, back and hips. Feel the muscles in your buttocks, thighs and calves go soft. Unclench your fingers, relax your jaw, free your ankles and your toes. Be aware of the fine current of electrical energy flowing through your lover's hands, through the fingertips. The more open you are to this energy, the more it will answer and resolve your own. Sometimes it may stir and release emotions such as joy or sadness. Simply allow your feelings to flow. The massage will leave you radiant, your mind clear and at peace.'

'What about pressure?' said Adam. 'How hard should I press?'

'If you use the muscles of your arms, hands, wrists and fingers to press, you will tire yourself and communicate the tension in your muscles to the receiver,' said Koriko. 'Instead, move smoothly from your belly, using the natural weight of your body. Think of yourself as pure energy, and of the massage as two energy fields interacting. Work with your mind to penetrate the body with healing intention rather than working with force.'

'Keep your spine straight so the energy can flow unhindered through all your chakras,' said Padmini, 'and stay well balanced – steady, even pressure is most effective and relaxing for both of you.'

'If the pressure is too strong,' said Marguerite, 'the receiver will tense up to resist, but too light a touch can be ticklish and annoying. The more deeply relaxed your partner is, the more deeply you can work. Just ask what feels good. The greater the pressure, the more it affects the muscles and blood vessels. The lighter the pressure, the more it affects the nerves – a light touch is good for gentle stimulation to begin and end.

'Areas that hold a lot of tension, like the upper

113

back, neck and shoulders, may need to be worked slowly and gently over several sessions. And be careful with the bones. Work with deep finger-pressure at either side of the spine and alongside and in between the other bones, not on top of them.'

'A word about rhythm,' said Koriko. 'Everything in the universe has its own rhythm – the orbits of the planets, the ebb and flow of the tides, the revolving seasons, the flow of the breath and the beat of the heart. Working to a rhythm feels calming and soothing, but feel free to change the rhythm or opt out of it as you need to. Use the heartbeat as your guide, or work to music that sounds as spacious as the breath and feels as though it could go on for ever.'

'Now to your repertoire of massage strokes,' said Padmini. 'Incorporate as many of these as you like into your massage, always making broad contact with an area of the body before you begin to work it in detail.

'Warm your hands before you begin. Shake them out with loose wrists and give them a vigorous rubbing. And warm the oil by spreading it between the palms of your hands before you apply it to the body.'

'The first stroke is *effleurage* – skimming,' said Marguerite. 'A slow flowing stroke with a broad flat palm. Start light, then lean into it with more pressure, turning it into a gliding stroke. As your hands skim in wide circles, fanning out and smoothing back across the skin, think of embracing, warmth, tranquillity, relaxation, protection. Work both hands together, or one rhythmically after the other, lapping like drifts of petals. Gather your lover's body between your palms. Keep your fingers together to conserve your energy.

'Make your touch slow and confident and your hand sensitive and listening. Appreciate the body you are touching with your eyes, and discover it with your hands as if you were a sculptor, interested in the anatomy beneath. Appreciate the softness of the skin, the warmth of the flesh, the shape of the muscles and bones; don't speak, apart from occasional murmurs of praise or endearment.'

'Working more deeply produces strokes that rub and pull, warming and invigorating the flesh,' said Padmini. 'Spread the palms to pull the flesh apart, up and down the back; across the back from side to side. Steady, gentle stretching. Use all these skimming, sliding and rubbing strokes across the back, the sides, upper chest, ribcage, arms and legs. They form the basis of your massage and, released from the formality of its structure, the basis of all sensual caressing.'

'When the flesh feels warmed and enlivened under your touch,' said Marguerite, 'move on to *petrissage*, or kneading. A deep movement that releases tension in the nerves, tissues and muscles and invigorates the blood. As if you were kneading bread, grasp the body tissues between your whole palms and fingers, pull gently away from the body then release. Work with generosity, not pinching, but plucking, amply squeezing and letting go. Use this technique to release the back of the neck and the shoulders. Work vigorously here and on the buttocks, but more gently on the abdomen, thighs and upper arms.'

'Rocking, rolling and shaking relax and tone the tissues', said Koriko. 'With one hand steadying the ankle, roll the flesh of the calf from side to side in your cupped palm. Or rock the hips or the ribcage gently between the flats of your two palms, one on either side of the body. Loose shaking between the palms on the thighs and buttocks can be energizing and dynamic when performed fast, or tantalizingly erotic when performed slowly and languorously. Shake the buttocks and legs inwards to relax them, and stretch and tease them out from the midline to arouse.'

Now Koriko demonstrated a vigorously stimulating technique. 'It calls for loose wrists and a rhythmic movement with alternate hands.' Working on Padmini's back, she showed them four variations. 'Pounding with loose fists, cupping with hollow palms, chopping with the sides of the hands and gentle slapping with open palms. These strokes are good all over the back, buttocks and backs of thighs. They feel invigorating, bringing blood to the surface and making the nerves tingle. They're also good for a standing back massage, like this one. As you see, Padmini bends over as I work down her back and straightens up again as I work back up it.

'After these vigorous strokes your partner will be ready for specific, deeper bodywork. To work the back, straddle the body so you can simultaneously treat the left and right sides. Starting at the base of the neck, drop your thumbs in at either side of the spine and work outwards to the shoulders – deeply satisfying to receive. Work rhythmically in lines either across or down the back, dropping your thumbs in, then wriggling them to resolve blockages and release tension.

'In the Oriental system of massage, we work specific points to free sexual energy. You can stimulate them by working in detail on the feet, around the ankles and above and below the knees at either side of the kneecap. Press gently with your fingertips or thumbs into the grooves and hollows, not directly on to the bones. On the front of the body, walk your fingers up and down the midline of the belly from the pubic bone to the navel, and work along the crease of the groin. There are many sexually sensitive points all over the inner upper thighs – caress them with your palms, or drum your fingertips all over the skin like falling rain. On the back, penetrate deeply with your thumbs along either side of the spine below the waist down to the crease of the buttocks, then along the inner cheeks of the buttocks, ending by feathering your fingers again all over the inner thighs.'

'Working all round the pubis with careful and detailed attention but not touching the genitals can feel very erotic', said Marguerite. 'Control the build-up of sexual tension by breaking off occasionally and incorporating more skimming and planing into the massage, reaching your palms up the midline of the body to the chest, then swooping back down the sides, gathering ever more energy to the genitals.

'Then slide one hand palm-up between the legs and under the buttocks, and press the other palm-down on the body above it, with the heel of the hand against the pubic bone and your fingers pointing towards the navel. Rest with your palms in this position, feeling the heat build between them. At this point you could end the massage and leave your partner covered with a light blanket to rest for a while. Quietly ask whether you should stop or go on.

'To continue the treatment, gently push the heels of your hands towards the upper body to stretch and stimulate the highly erogenous flesh between them. Then hold one hand still and rock the other, first slowly, then faster. Repeat with the other hand.

'Now you are ready to touch the sex organs,' said Padmini. 'But remember that this is a massage and don't be tempted away from its formalized structure. Take more oil in your palms and rub it in well, all over your hands and fingers, until they are warm and slippery.' She turned to Adam. 'When you massage Eve, begin with the first two fingers of each hand touching at the perineum, the muscular bridge between the genitals and the anus, and gently push them up and forward, round the outer lips of her yoni, to meet just inside the pubic bone. Stroke back and forwards along this path many times, describing with silky fingers the tall oval shape with the pointed ends that is the symbol of the yoni. Then slide your fingertips inside the outer lips and repeat the action. Stroke very lightly and rhythmically, up the inner lips and over the rosy bead of the clitoris where they join at the top; trail the weight of your fingertips across the sensitive flesh as if stroking gold leaf without tearing it. Follow this inner oval with your fingertips many times until all the energies of her body are highly stimulated. Eve may enter an altered state of consciousness or experience spontaneous orgasm, but this is not the aim of the exercise.

'When she is highly charged with sexual energy, her yoni is red and swollen, her face flushed, her lips are parted and her glowing eyes are half closed, drowsy with desire, touch the fully engorged clitoris once with the pad of your thumb, as if leaving a thumbprint. Then release and circle the clitoris very gently many times with your fingertip. This action is called Stirring the Fire. Again, this may cause Eve to spiral into spontaneous orgasm as it sends sexual energy radiating to every part of the body.

'End Eve's massage by cupping her yoni in the palm of your hand. Press firmly with the heel of the hand against the perineum. Rock the yoni gently under your hand, to still and comfort it. Sweep both hands from the pubis up the midline of the chest and down the sides, continuing right down the thighs to the knees. Move lightly up the insides of the legs and continue up the midline of the body, making this double oval several times to unify the body and spread and calm the energies. Place one palm on Eve's belly and the other on the heart chakra between her breasts. Let them rest there a while as you send cherishing thoughts through your palms. Then lift your hands so lightly from her body that she does not feel them leave it. Cover her and let her rest.'

Padmini turned to Eve. 'You can perform the final sequence of the erotic massage on Adam whether his lingam is erect or not. Either way, the massage will tone and energize his whole system and help him with ejaculation control. Oil and warm your hands well. If he doesn't have an erection, take the lingam in your left hand and hold it back against his belly, as if it were erect. Cradle your hand beneath it, holding the head lightly between your thumb and forefinger. Cup the testicles in your right hand to warm them. Rest in this position while you breathe deeply, sending the warmth of your breath flooding into your hands. Move your right hand up to cover the lingam, so that you are holding it still between both hands, like a prayer. Then with the thumb of your right hand, stroke lightly from the perineum, between the testicles and up the midline of the shaft to the head. Repeat this stroke softly many times. The lingam may erect, but there is no pressure for this to happen.

'If the lingam is not erect, perform Stirring the Fire by circling with your fingertip the midpoint on the wrinkled frenulum, the point at which the fore-skin is attached to the glans. Circle it several times, then lay the lingam gently on his belly and cover it briefly with both hands before sweeping them up his chest and back down his sides to his thighs in a generous circling motion to smooth and settle his energies.

'If his lingam is erect, hold it in your left hand against his belly, with your hand beneath it and the head held lightly between your thumb and fore-finger. With the thumb and forefinger of your right hand, stroke up the midline of the shaft and down the side, round the testicle, up the midline and down the other side, and so on, stroking in this long figure of eight many times. The massage will be most effective if you keep to the instructions!

To perform Stirring the Fire on an erect lingam, draw back the foreskin as far as you can, holding the lingam pointing up from his body in your fist. Then with your right index finger, circle around the corona, the collar of the glans, many times. Each of these rhythmic stroking and circling movements is like a meditation. The massage is unlikely to trigger ejaculation, and neither is that its purpose. As with the yoni massage, this sequence will flood Adam's body with sexual energy and leave him feeling powerful and relaxed. When you have finished circling the corona, lay the lingam back on Adam's belly. Close your hands around it briefly in the prayer position. Then swoop your hands up his chest, down his sides and over his thighs in a generous circle to resolve and settle his energies. Place one palm on his belly and the other on his heart chakra. Let them rest there as you send adoring thoughts through your palms. Then lift your hands so lightly from his body that he does not feel them leave it. Cover him and let him rest.'

'You can *feel* the difference the massage has made,' said Koriko quietly, breaking the peaceful silence that had descended. 'Hold your hand flat and relaxed just above your lover's body and move it gently from head to toe, like a scanner. You will feel the thrilling tingle of electric energy released by your touch.'

SCROLL 3

Sipping Nectar

❧

The Courtesans' Parchment

Running like a golden thread through the myriad customs that surround kissing is an undisputed belief in the emotional nourishment of the lovers' kiss.

EW CARESSES ARE AS RICH IN SUBTLETY and emotional intensity as the kiss. From the tender brushing of cheeks to the parting of the lips, the urgent meeting of tongues and the passionate exploration of each other's mouths, every kiss between lovers develops its own original, spontaneously evolving plot. The kiss roams thrillingly through many degrees of excitement, even to orgasm.

The first deep kiss marks the awakening of sexuality and encapsulates the promise of all that is to come. The folk tales of many countries tell how the meeting of mouths has the power to transform lives and release the radiant beauty trapped within.

The kiss at the end of the fairy tale is the gateway to happiness for the simple reason that the pleasure of kissing is addictive, promising a future filled with erotic delights. The ancients knew that the intoxicating secret of the kiss lay in its chemistry, the tasting on the breath, lips and tongue of an aphrodisiac elixir unique to each couple. And modern science has confirmed that the thirst for kisses is fuelled by the hormones and bonding chemicals kissing releases in the mouth.

Deep-mouth kissing induces a rush of fresh saliva. In the East, this precious nectar was rightly hailed as the source of erotic nourishment of the kiss, a well that never runs dry. According to Taoist and Tantric texts, the most nourishing and voluptuous way to kiss is to suck at the lips of the beloved, and gently to nibble at the tongue to make the nectar flow sweet and exquisite, more delicious than the finest honey. The beloved's tongue can then be rolled into a tube that the lover takes completely in his mouth to suck nectar from all its surfaces. Of the three sets of salivary glands in the mouth, the sublingual glands beneath the tongue secrete the least, but this type of saliva is the most highly prized, being particularly fragrant and fresh.

The aphrodisiac chemicals in saliva have only recently been discovered by Western science, yet the Chinese knew five thousand years ago that the love juices of the mouth contained the essence of the lover's sexuality. In the case of a woman, the essence is described as *yin*, which means that it has the power to nourish, strengthen and satisfy a man, over and over again. The male essence is *yang*: it energizes a woman and fires all her passions. Yin and yang complement and balance each other; the nectar of the kiss not only heightens erotic excitement, but through its nourishing qualities, improves the health and promotes long life.

A kiss communicates more intimately than genital sex because it requires full dedication and commitment. And because the chemical match created by the kiss is unique, passionate kissing tends to be monotropic – instinctively dedicated to just one adored person. Thus a courtesan will kiss on the mouth only the man she loves, and deep erotic kissing leaves a crumbling relationship long before penetration ceases.

The kisses of others are deliciously revealing. The secretly glimpsed deep–mouth kiss is the confirmation of a full and free sexual life, standing for what we are not allowed to see but can only imagine. So flagrant is the link between deep–mouth kissing and sex that in some parts of the world to be seen kissing the mouth of another's wife or husband constitutes proof of adultery.

Knowing the seductive and binding power of a kiss, men and women have always sought to invite attention to their mouths. Men do it with beards and moustaches; women find ways of emphasizing their lips. Since the days of ancient Egypt, female lips have been painted to look fuller and redder in imitation of the lips of the genitals, when swollen with excitement. In Sudan it was the tradition for women to tattoo their lower lips to accentuate the bruising caused by the erotic delights of biting and sucking them. In tribal societies across Africa and South America women have long worn wooden lip plates. Among the Surma and Mursi peoples of Ethiopia, the girls with the largest lip plates command the highest bride prices. The process of enlargement is started by inserting a coin-sized plug into a slit in the lower lip, then gradually replacing it with larger and larger discs. The girl looks irresistibly kissable to her lover, and when she takes out the lip plate in the privacy of their room he will ecstatically nibble and suck at her over-large lower lip.

How did kissing originate? The world's first word for kiss, in the ancient Indo-European language of Sanskrit, is *cusati*, meaning 'he sucks'. In ancient Egypt there was a word that meant both 'kiss' and 'eat'. Psychologists claim that the kiss harks back to sucking the maternal breast. The first sight of the breast, the first sensation of sucking, the first feed, form the foundation of all future expectations and experiences of comfort and satisfaction, and the basis for all life's erotic bonds. But anthropologists say the origin of the kiss lies in another sort of feeding, a method of weaning in which the mother passes chewed food from her own mouth into her baby's mouth – and both use tongues. Kiss-feeding was common in ancient Greece and is still used today by hunter-gatherers in the rainforests of Venezuela.

The instincts of hunger and love combine to create a blurring in the imagination between kissing, biting and eating. The desire to devour and consume the beloved to merge souls in ecstatic possession was enacted literally by some primitive societies. Anthropophagy was a custom in which a beautiful young man was slaughtered and eaten as a god. The belief was that by devouring the flesh of the god, it was possible to assimilate his divine qualities and make him live again through the life of the one who ate him. Many saviour gods have been symbolically cannibalized, including Osiris and Jesus. Those who eat the body and drink the blood as bread and wine will be imbued with divine truth and redemption. In the erotic kiss–bite of the vampire, the story is upended. The vampire sucks vital fluid from his victim and imparts his haunted nocturnal nature to the sleeping un-fortunate, who must in turn survive by kiss–biting new victims. In the erotic world of gods and vampires, devouring and being devoured are the same as being reborn. In the erotic world of mortals, kissing provides the same spiritual transformation.

If kissing, tasting and eating are all linked in the sensual imagination, so are kissing, smelling and breathing. The Taoists had a practice called sniff-kissing, in which they inhaled aphrodisiac essences from the beloved's body, and the ancient Egyptians must have known it too, because they had a word that meant both 'kiss' and 'smell'. The Khyoungthas, who live in the foothills of the Himalayas, kiss by pressing the nose to the cheek of the beloved, then inhaling while smacking the lips. Among Mongols, Native Americans and Eskimos there is a tradition of kissing by rubbing noses to inhale the breath of the loved one, and the Chittagongs of Bangladesh actually say not 'kiss me' but 'smell me', as they breathe in their partner's odour.

Smell is the sense of memory and desire. To inhale the lover's breath is to breathe in the beloved body through one's mouth and nose, and to possess it instantly, in its most secret essence, across many subtle layers of erotic memory. A steamy kiss opens the pores of the forehead; pearls of sweat release aphrodisiac pheromones to mingle with the breath. When a woman kisses a man she often raises her arms to cup his face in her hands. His face is close to her armpits; her body heat carries her musky sexual odours to his nose. The Tantrics say that if during a kiss a man draws into his right nostril the breath from a woman's left nostril, making a perfect circle of breathing between them, the couple will enjoy lasting love and devotion.

The exchange of breath in the mouth-to-mouth kiss is poetically believed to mingle souls. At a medieval marriage mass the union was sealed with such a kiss, after which the souls of bride and groom were considered to be one. And to die with your lover's kiss on your lips was the ideal of medieval Courtly Love, for it was the gateway to paradise.

Running like a golden thread through the myriad customs that surround kissing is an undisputed belief in the emotional nourishment of the lovers' kiss. It creates a deep bond of sensuality and a vision of the erotic that is at once breathtakingly thrilling and comfortingly secure. Understanding that passionate kissing was the key to the health of the lovers and their relationship, the ancients studied, developed and refined the art, devising many imaginative erotic variations to keep lovers kissing.

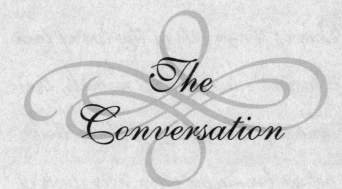

The
Conversation

One of the secrets of the art of love

is to move two steps forwards, then

one step back, to cool the ardour

before bringing on a new flush of

even more intense heat . . .

THE COURTESANS' PARTY CONTINUED THEIR
journey on horseback. Crossing a
magical terrain flooded by moonlight,
they followed a stream that rushed and tumbled
brightly over smooth boulders until they reached
its source. The spring gushed from the rock to fill a
deep pool brimful, before cascading down the hill-
side. Adam and Eve and the three courtesans
gathered in a circle round the pool. As they leaned
over towards the cool water they saw their silvered
reflections dance on its inky surface, and in the
centre high above them the mysterious pale disc of
the moon. Then, following Marguerite's example,
they cupped their hands to receive the sparkling

water from the source and drank deeply. The water tasted of the history of the rocks from which it sprang, alive and rich in minerals.

'In France we have a saying that lovers can live on kisses and cool water', said Marguerite, taking a last sip and savouring its refreshing purity. 'And now we have drunk from the spring, let us sit down and talk.' They made themselves comfortable on a bank of fragrant herbs, and under the starry sky, to the chirping of cicadas in the still warmth of the night their moonlit discussion began. 'Your third step on the path to the Seventh Heaven is devoted to exploring every nuance of the erotic pleasure of kissing', said Marguerite. 'To feel the real thrill of the kiss, indulge in kissing for its own sake, instead of as a prelude to sex.'

'As you have read, the kiss is the eternal spark of love', said Padmini, 'so keep your love on fire by always parting and greeting with a kiss. How right the gypsies are, when they say that a kiss is worth nothing until divided between two! So look intently into each other's eyes as your faces move closer, then shut your eyes and put your whole being into your lips as they touch your lover's mouth. Forget everything else while you kiss. For as long as it takes to breathe in the scent of your lover's skin, let four lips together be your entire world. A kiss of parting and greeting is made with the mouth almost closed, but just the merest touch of the warm, moist inner skin sends the secret message of desire.'

'A public kiss to the palm of your beloved's hand would be an unusual intimacy in your culture,' Koriko said to Adam. 'Apply your closed lips to the centre of the palm. In acupuncture this is a vital point that leads straight to the heart and the breath, and can be used in both calming and exciting the emotions. The pressure in your lips can transmit much more than this chaste kiss seems to say. Apply this kiss to the heart points along the crease of Eve's even more sensitive inner wrist, and she will experience a mixture of the formal and the erotic that is purely Japanese. And in the bedroom, a more lascivious version of this kiss will send a thrill all the way up her arm and through her nipple, down to the Cinnabar Field of her yoni. Lick lavishly across the inner wrist. Trail your tongue to the middle of the palm and tantalize the sensitive spot right in the centre with the tip. Run the tongue up the middle finger, taking it completely into your mouth and sucking vigorously; let the fingertip fall out of your mouth with a slurp.

'But I am getting carried away,' Koriko apologized, fanning herself delicately. 'Before we discuss erotic kissing, there are preparations to be made. First, make sure your mouth is ready for the kiss. Some women like to kiss a man with a beard, but stubble can rasp against delicate skin and make it sore. My lovers always shaved their beards very closely so their kisses were like silk. That was the custom in those days. And pay careful attention to hygiene. The scent of a lover's breath and mouth, both out-side and inside, is highly arousing, so take care that your mouth tastes fresh and sweet like the spring. Scrape your tongue, floss your teeth and use a toothbrush after every meal.'

'A toothbrush!' said Marguerite. 'But you had a fashion for blacking your teeth!'

'Blackened teeth in my culture were indeed beautiful,' Koriko agreed with a bow, 'though the custom had all but died out by the beginning of the twentieth century. The black teeth disappeared like the night against the red-painted lips and the white-painted face, making the mouth look bigger and redder.'

'We cleaned our teeth with splinters of wood,' said Marguerite, 'and scraped our tongues with twigs, then rubbed them with a cloth. I chewed parsley to sweeten my breath.'

'I cracked fragrant fennel seeds between my teeth to sweeten mine,' said Padmini.

'We exercised our mouths to keep our lips soft and pliant for kissing,' said Koriko, and to their amusement she demonstrated an exercise called

Dragon Lips. 'Watch yourself in the mirror as you roll the lips inwards past the teeth, then part them as widely as you can and extend them above and below, as if breathing out fire. Then purse them, pushing them forwards as far as they will go to blow out the fire. Keep rolling your lips like this until they are warm and tingling.

'Geishas performed this routine several times on rising in the morning, but kissing itself is the best exercise to keep you looking young and vibrant. All the facial muscles are involved in a kiss, and as the kiss progresses, the breathing grows more urgent, flushing the body cells with oxygen; the pulse accelerates, boosting the circulation and flooding the body with exhilarating warmth. The lips engorge with blood, reddening and swelling like other erectile body tissue – the genitals and nipples. Hormones surge in the blood, lifting the spirits to euphoria.'

'When you are ready to kiss,' said Padmini, 'look into each other's eyes. A deep look can be almost unbearably arousing – the anticipation of a kiss can hold you in a spell that turns your insides to liquid and makes your skin crackle with eroticism. Cup your lover's head in your hands as if drinking from a flower. Instinctively you tilt your heads so your lips can meet. Close your eyes to immerse yourself in your other senses. Inhale the scent of your lover's skin and breath. Brush cheeks; rub noses, gently. Find each other's lips. Allow the lips to part. Inhale the scented warmth of your lover's breath. Touch tongues, move them against each other, pushing, sliding, tasting, probing deep into your lover's mouth.'

'Why is it called French kissing?' asked Eve.

'Legend has it that deep-mouth kissing was enjoyed for hours on end by the fishing people of Brittany', said Marguerite. 'While waiting for the tide so they could set to sea, they occupied their time by thrusting their tongues in and out of their lovers' mouths in imitation of the ebb and flow of the tide. The same kiss is called in Latin *suavium*, because of its unending smoothness.'

'In India we call this kiss the battle of the tongues,' said Padmini. 'Dart inside your lover's mouth with your tongue all hot, slippery and elastic, and explore. Be the kisser or the kissed, or you can both thrust and probe together. Massage the roof of the mouth, work over and under the tongue, flick your tongue over the teeth, like a dance. Just when you think the kiss is ending, change pace and the excitement rises again so you feel it scorch like lightning up your belly. The kiss lingers, then leaps on, then slows again, then your lover moves away to ravish your throat and neck, returning more hungrily than ever to your mouth.'

'Kissing is addictive, as you have read,' said Koriko, turning to Adam, 'because saliva contains hormones and potent bonding chemicals. Sipping the nectar of the mouth increases desire; drinking from the precious fountain of the tongue promotes health and longevity. In the Orient we say that the tongue is the sprout of the heart, meaning it conveys all the heart's emotions. Use your tongue with all the consciousness of your heart to stimulate her tongue, then savour the flow of honeyed love juices in her mouth and drink them as an elixir. The taste buds sensitive to sweetness are near the tip of the tongue. So tease the roof of her mouth with the tip of your tongue and let it slide around the back teeth on both sides, where the nectar gushes forth. Sweep the floor of her mouth inside the teeth and push your tongue repeatedly at the root of her tongue to release more juices. This stimulation will produce a rich flow of nectar in both your mouths. Gulp this heady aphrodisiac from the source.'

'One of the secrets of the art of love is to move two steps forwards, then one step back, to cool the ardour before bringing on a new flush of even more intense heat,' said Marguerite. 'So after the French kiss, retreat to the lip brush. Part your lips. Brush them lightly across your lover's skin, barely touch-ing. Breathe out slowly, so your lover feels a slice of hot air inside two warm, dry lips. Try this kiss around and over the mouth. Pull back swiftly as she tries to trap your tongue in a full kiss – and brush your lips away and across her throat.'

'Kissing is like music and needs changes of mood and pace,' said Koriko. 'Embrace Eve from behind and bury your face in the fragrance of her hair. Lift her hair and tenderly kiss the nape of her neck, a point of exquisite vulnerability that Japanese men find particularly alluring in their women. As you begin to loosen her clothes, inhale her perfume. In the Orient we say that a woman has Ten Fragrances. We inhale these fragrances in the sniff-kiss, which we also use to breathe in the scent of a newborn baby. The Ten Fragrances are Eve's hair, her bosom, her cheeks, neck, tongue, lips, fingers, feet, the flower of her sex, and her entire body. The erotic swoon induced by the sniff-kiss is so potent that a poem about the Ten Fragrances written by an empress of the Liao dynasty was used as evidence of adultery against her, and caused her tragic death.'

'In India we also love the sniff-kiss,' said Padmini,

'especially if the lover's body is perfumed lightly with crushed jasmine or tuberose to enhance its sexual aroma. Begin by deeply inhaling Eve's breath, then nudge your nose against her eyelids, cheeks and neck and continue the scented pilgrimage up the peak and down the valley of her breasts.'

'The sounds of love are highly erotic', said Marguerite. 'A kiss sounds like eating luscious fruit. A voluptuous sigh is evidence of sheer delight. Deep inhalation follows, bringing vitality surging around the body so the heart beats more strongly, and the senses sharpen. Then there are the guttural noises, deep moans, little purring sounds in the throat. You may want to laugh with happiness as your mood moves from passion to elation. Or you may find tears of emotion drenching your cheeks. Whisper words of endearment that tell what you're feeling as you kiss.'

'Warm your partner's skin by puffing little hot kisses just above it', said Padmini, 'as if blowing smoke rings from a hookah. There is no contact except with small explosions of hot air. Then move in closer for the vibrating kiss. Put your slightly parted lips to your lover's skin and breathe a "vvv" sound through them, making them vibrate. This is another very warming kiss.'

'Try a luscious gliding kiss along your lover's sensitive inner arms and legs, or down his spine,' said Marguerite, turning to Eve. 'These areas are too large to be lubricated with saliva, which in any case evaporates and cools the skin, so use almond oil, with its delicate nutty taste. Smooth it in well with your fingers, then suck and slide your lips from the inner wrist right up the arm. Try this in one sweep, or bring the tongue into play, twirling it in loop over loop. Working towards the centre of the body creates a crescendo of desire.'

'Press the tip of the tongue firmly against a point that is just to the side of your erotic target, such as the outer corner of the open mouth,' said Padmini. 'Press strongly, dancing the tip, then allow it to suddenly fall into the mouth, as if by mistake, and quickly withdraw it. This is the tantalizing kiss.'

'I love to kiss the ear,' said Koriko, 'thrusting and probing with my tongue tip into the centre. The ear has over a hundred acupuncture points and they can all be enlivened and massaged by swirling your tongue around its shell-like curves. There are three love points you should take care to press – they all lie around the point on the earlobe that a woman stimulates naturally when she puts on her earrings. These points relax the muscles while stimulating the ovaries and the release of hormones. You can work them by sucking and nibbling the earlobe.'

'Are there any other secret places to kiss that will give Eve special pleasure?' asked Adam.

'Try licking her armpit, and pressing your tongue along the fine skin of the crease where her thigh joins her abdomen,' said Marguerite. 'Try lapping like a cat behind her knee and in the crook of her elbow.'

'Padmini, what kisses can you teach us from the *Kamasutra*?' Eve asked.

'Kisses that suck and nibble the lips,' said Padmini. 'First, suck Adam's upper lip into your mouth. As you pull on the lip run your tongue along the join of his mouth and gum and appreciate its sweetness. Now press with your fingers to squeeze his lower lip into a red ball. Use "blunt teeth" to hold, tug, and gnaw softly at the juicy lip. Finally grasp both his lips inside your own and suck them.

'Then there's the love bite. My lovers sometimes used to bite my neck, here where it joins my shoulders, as a trophy of our secret assignation. If you are bitten in the heat of passion, you are less likely to feel the pain. A love bite leaves the imprint of the teeth and a dark purplish bruise between them. If you want to try it, build up to it gradually. Once your lover is lost in wild abandon, sink your teeth into his flesh, pressing hard without cutting the skin, and suck powerfully between your teeth. The force of the suck brings the blood to the surface of the skin, creating a bruise. The next day he can wear a scarf to hide the mark – or flaunt it with pride.'

'You Indians are barbaric, Padmini!' said Marguerite. 'I should hate to be bitten. Have you no more sensual kisses for us?'

'Yes, indeed,' said Padmini. 'Here is a kiss called watermelon nibbling. Squeeze the ample flesh of your lover's hips and buttocks towards you with both hands and gently nibble as you suck, lick, and salivate, as if you were dissolving the flesh of a watermelon in your mouth with the juices running down your face.

'Or try a kiss feast, feeding your lover luscious, ripe strawberries from your mouth – do it in the bath where you can revel in the mess and laughter. Scatter nasturtiums and marigolds on the water. Give him a sumptuous face massage with still fruity papaya and mango skins, then lick and suck away the juice. Tease your lover with chocolate kisses; feed him oysters from your lips. Sip champagne from melon skins and pass it from your mouth to his. Slurp it from his navel!'

'So many ideas!' said Eve. 'If you had to give just

one piece of advice on kissing, what would it be?'

'To forget all about the techniques we have discussed and to lose yourself in the pleasure of the moment', said Marguerite. 'To be instinctive, inventive and adventurous. To adore your lover with your mouth, lips and tongue, and to feel adored in return.'

SCROLL 4

The Hills of Paradise

❧

The Courtesans' Parchment

The miracle of the breast and the celestial nature of life's vital drink is celebrated in the myths of many cultures.

THE EROTIC FASCINATION OF THE BREAST cannot be disentangled from deep longings for the lost paradise of being an infant in a warm and milky embrace. Behind every uplifting vision of the breasts (as we mentioned when we talked of kissing), lie the first sight, the first sensation, the first feed, which form the foundation of all life's expectations and experiences of comfort and satisfaction, and the basis for all life's erotic bonds. So the breasts are an irresistible magnet for the imagination and, particularly in Western culture where babies are weaned early and the breasts are hidden, there is a need to look and devour with the eyes, even through clothes.

The shape of the breasts is unique to every woman; even each individual breast is subtly different, as symmetry is not a feature of breasts any more than it is of faces. Girlish breasts are high and round and far apart, but when they mature, some breasts slide shyly down the body, while others swell in maternal splendour. There are breasts shaped like apples, mangoes, melons. Some point up, others outwards. Nipples may be thick, dark and stubbily erect or pale and flat. The areola may be small and crinkly or smooth and wide, as if spread broadly around the nipple with the tongue.

The breast is the source of the most tender love and kindness. The universal character of breasts is their generous compassion, the life–giving role they have played in the history of human survival. The earliest known idols – among them the Venus of Willendorf, a small limestone figurine believed to be twenty–five thousand years old – honour the power of the breast. The Venus is endowed with massively swelling bosoms as well as a vast stomach and rolling buttocks. Her ample curves promised fertility and plenty in a world where starvation always threatened. Prehistoric women desperate to feed their babies may well have prayed to such ample idols to fill their breasts with milk.

In Egypt there is a statue of the goddess–queen Isis breast–feeding Horus. Sitting on the lap of the goddess was the same as mounting the throne, and to drink milk from her breast was to be recognized as her heir and made immortal. However, the most astonishing example of breast power is the Greek statue of Artemis of Ephesus, goddess of nurture, fertility and birth. Her whole torso is covered in breasts, about twenty of them. Her arms are spread in an invitation to drink from her abundant and everlasting supply of milk.

The miracle of the breast and the celestial nature of life's vital drink is celebrated in the myths of many cultures. Look out of the window at the night sky full of stars twinkling in the inky blackness and listen to the story of how ancient peoples all over the world imagined they got there. Like the Egyptians, the Greeks told of the milk of immortality – and how anyone who drank from the breast of the goddess would become divine. So when Zeus wanted his mortal son Hercules to become a god, he put him to the breast of his consort Hera while she lay asleep. But the youngster sucked so vigorously that the queen of the goddesses woke up and, realizing he was not her child, thrust him away. As she did so, the shining droplets of her milk cascaded like a fountain into the velvet darkness of the firmament to hang there as stars, which is how the Milky Way came into being. That shimmering cloudy swirl of infinite numbers of stars is our galaxy, and 'galaxy' itself comes from two words, *gala* and *lac*, which both mean milk.

Everywhere the goddess's immortal star milk formed curds to create worlds. From India to Scandinavia the Moon–Cow goddess was recognized as the mother of the world and the one who gave nourishment to the spirits of the stars. Today there are still people in India who believe that the universe was curdled from the milk of the Cow, which is why that animal is revered as sacred. According to Japanese tradition the first landmasses clumped together when the gods churned the Sea of Milk, which went *koworokoworo* ('curdlecurdle'). The early people of the Bible lands thought that human bodies too were curdled from primeval milk. Job asks, 'Hast thou not poured me out as milk, and curdled me like cheese?'

In Egypt the cow-headed goddess Hathor, the bringer of love and joy, created the Milky Way as a river of her own milk, which she called 'the Nile in the Sky'. She offered her breasts with both hands and those she suckled drank in with her milk a secret soul name, a *ren*, which would transport them safely into the afterlife. This magic name was the same as rennet, an enzyme found in the stomach of a calf that was used in antiquity as it is today to curdle milk and turn it into a dessert called junket.

Like a *gala*, a *junket* came to mean a feast or festival, a magical transformation of the everyday. Milk has always signified abundance and celebration – the land flowing with milk and honey is a paradise and its emblem is a cornucopia, a cow's horn of plenty pouring out all the bounty of the earth.

The
Conversation

In the language of alchemy the heart is the chakra of transformations, the crucible in which the purifying fire turns base materials to gold.

ADAM AND EVE AWOKE FROM READ-ing the fourth parchment scroll to find themselves reclining on a soft bank of fragrant herbs. It was night. Below them in the valley a fire blazed in the darkness. As they made their way down the hill towards it they recognized the three women basking in its warmth and ran to meet them. Padmini welcomed them.

'The fourth step on your journey to the Seventh Heaven celebrates the rich and beautiful bounty of the breasts,' she said, inviting them to sit by the fire. 'Nestling between the breasts is the wellspring of our emotions, the whirling vortex of the heart chakra.' She pressed her hand on the place. 'The three chakras above the heart belong to the heavens and the three below it to the earth. So the breast is the place where heaven and earth meet and all contradictions are resolved. In the language of alchemy the heart is the chakra of trans-formations, the crucible in which the purifying fire turns base materials to gold. The breast is where the energies of body and mind meet and the sexual opens out into the spiritual realm. The transforming fire of the heart chakra is love.

'In Buddhist and Hindu practices there is an ancient meditation that brings the fire of the heart chakra into the hands. It is very simple and goes like this: sit quietly with eyes closed, your palms resting lightly on your thighs, and become aware of your breath flowing in and out. Don't alter your breathing, just be aware of it. Then start to breathe in deeply to your belly. Fold your hands over your belly and feel it rise and fall. Once a rhythm is well established, put your palms flat against your ribcage, with fingers pointing in to the midline of your chest. Breathe in to the belly, pause, and breathe further in, allowing your breath to push out the ribcage. Exhale. Inhale in two stages again and feel your hands being forced further apart. After several breaths like this, move one palm to your heart chakra and rest the other on your thigh. Continue deep-breathing, adding a third stage of inhalation, feeling the breath rise to fill your upper chest. Exhale. Continue to breathe the three-stage breath and you will feel the point at the centre of your palm flush with heat at the cusp of the breath just before you exhale. As you breathe, imagine your heart and your hands opening and radiating love and tenderness towards yourself, your beloved and all other beings.'

'I have heard that meditation is good for the heart,' said Adam, 'but I have never known how to begin.'

'There are two types of meditation,' said Marguerite: 'with and without focus. With focus is the easier. But still the mind gets diverted and carried away by the trivia of everyday, thoughts and feelings flit across the consciousness, lists of things that need attending to, cares that work round and round – all this disturbs the mind like ripples on a pond. Stilling the mind is difficult. But don't be hard on yourself. When you notice the mind is wandering, bring it back. If you can experience pure peace untrammelled by thought even for a moment, it will leave you refreshed, revived and centred. Meditation develops a sense of security in connectedness, a freedom in being at one, and it allows you to flow like water around the obstacles in life's path instead of hitting them head–on. It is a letting go that embraces all experience, all of life with an open and generous heart.

'Perhaps you wish to meditate on the loveliness of Eve's breasts. Find a quiet time and place. Sit and focus your mind on the beauty of her breasts, and the emotions they inspire in you, bringing your attention gradually to a single point, the very essence of Eve's breasts. Let your mind relax and be still, empty of other things. Open yourself to the object of your contemplation with the wonder of a child. Let it fill your entire consciousness until you and the object merge and become one, so deep is your awareness and your experience of it. Use the power of engagement that you discover in meditation to help you in your daily life, so that you perform even the most mundane tasks with freshness and calm, remaining focused on what you are doing instead of living an unsatisfactory else-where-life in your mind.

'Bring this same meditative awareness to Eve's breasts when you caress them.'

Koriko turned to Eve. 'I have a physical exercise for you that also has spiritual benefits,' she said, 'a traditional routine for enhancing the beauty of your breasts. It stimulates the production of hormones and helps nursing mothers produce milk. Every morning on waking, I rub my palms together to warm them, then massage both breasts simul-taneously, bringing my hands in a circle up between my breasts and over the top of them to the sides. I do this thirty-six times, then reverse and circle thirty-six times in the other direction. It feels beautiful, calming and nourishing.

'I learned this exercise from an old but youthfully beautiful woman with whom I studied for a time in Taiwan, Madame Bo. She was a White Tigress, a member of an ancient Taoist sect dating back three thousand years. The White Tigresses are women highly disciplined in meditation and energy exercises who dedicate their lives to sexual practices. Their aim is to harness the most powerful energy of human experience – sexual energy – and apply it to the pursuit of health, youthfulness, longevity and spiritual immortality. The Tigresses devised a whole massage sequence to firm the breasts and keep them healthy. It increases sexual energy, safeguards against the formation of lumps and tumours, and regulates the secretions of the endocrine glands. Women who practise it every day find that their periods become regular and less painful, with reduced flow. Some Tigresses practised until their periods stopped altogether, using it as a natural method of contraception.'

'How can massaging the breasts stop a woman's periods?' asked Adam.

'The massage acts like the sucking of the infant at the breast, which also has a contraceptive effect,' said Koriko. 'It would hardly be a reliable contraceptive, of course.'

'I would love to regulate my periods,' said Eve. 'Could you teach me the exercise?'

Koriko bowed. 'The exercise is called the Deer. I perform it naked, sitting on the floor. My room is warm and private and I sit cross-legged with one heel pressed against my yoni to stop sexual energy escaping. (If you can't get your heel into that position, put a ball between your heel and the yoni, so that you can feel the pressure.) Then I rub my hands together to warm them, and place one over each breast with the nipples protruding between my thumb and index fingers. I rest like this for a moment, relaxing my shoulders and enjoying the sensation of the warmth from my hands spreading into my breasts, then I begin to rotate my breasts gently, moving them upwards and outwards forty-eight times. Once this sequence is complete, I perform the same circling movements, but this time instead of rotating the breasts, I stimulate the nipples and areolae with four fingers only. This also I do forty-eight times. In the third part of the exercise I repeat the circling movement, but with just my fingers massaging my whole breasts. Finally, I take the nipples between the thumb and index finger of each hand. I breathe in deeply to my belly, pulling the nipple gently outwards, then exhale and release. I repeat this pulling and releasing twenty-four times.

'To make the treatment even more powerful,' Koriko added, 'I finish with a breathing exercise. Still sitting cross-legged, I draw the breath in through my nose to my chest, and imagine it flooding warmly into my breasts, expanding and enlivening them. As I draw in the breath, I pull up the muscles of the perineum and abdomen, contracting and locking the pelvic floor. I hold my breath and the contraction to a count of ten. Then I release, expelling the breath powerfully through my mouth. White Tigresses perform this exercise forty-eight times, but it takes quite a while to build up to this number. Perhaps you should start with twelve a day, then increase to twenty-four, and so on.'

Marguerite laid a gentle hand on Eve's arm. 'And now let us discuss how to enhance the erotic power of the breasts,' she said. 'The cleavage, that heavenly valley between two rolling hills, is a magnet to the male eye. Make the most of it. Dangle a jewelled pendant between the breasts to transfix and tantalize the gaze. Even a choker of chaste pearls draws the attention subtly downwards, allowing the imagination to do the rest. Perfume your breasts with a dab of oil of rose – it's the scent of the heart chakra. I have known women paint their exposed upper breasts with delicate blue veins, and shadow the cleavage with makeup. The deeper the plunge, the more exciting the incomplete view of nudity. The breasts themselves are accomplices in the erotic concealment – simultaneously thrust into view and coyly crowding together to hide as much of each other as they can.

Try the art of teasing with any cleavage on the body – low-cut shoes deliciously reveal the cleft between the toes, a bent arm invites the eye to the intriguing crook of the elbow. The tease was taken to its limits by the women of ancient Egypt, who bared their breasts completely, except for the smallest concealment of artfully gilding or rouging their nipples, and by the ladies of fifteenth-century France, whose daring *décolletage* revealed nipples pierced with diamonds and small decorative chains. In a man's fantasy the "yes–no" message of the tease is more enticing than complete submission because of the irresistible challenge it imposes.'

'The breasts have been thrust brazenly forward and then primly concealed in a flirtatious cycle of teasing throughout the history of fashion,' said Koriko. 'The invention of the brassiere itself hid an erotic secret. At the beginning of the eighth century in China, a favourite concubine of Emperor Tang Hsuan–tsung had a passionate affair with one of his generals. One night the general made love to the concubine with too much abandon, biting her as he sucked her breasts, and scratching her tender flesh with his nails. Fearing for her life if her secret was discovered, the concubine consulted with her maid and together they sewed a bandeau of red silk to hide the guilty wound. The Emperor found the style so enchanting for the delights it concealed, and the uplifting power this had on his imagination, that he asked her to wear it often. The bandeau–brassiere soon became a fashion among all the Emperor's concubines; some were even embroidered with erotic scenes.'

Marguerite turned to Eve. 'Your lingerie is best kept hidden, a secret between you and your lover,' she said confidentially. 'But pay attention to the profile your bra creates beneath your clothes, which can make all the difference in the world to your figure and the way you feel about your body. When you choose a bra, enlist the help of a trained expert who will ensure a perfect fit. Too many women, I have noticed, choose a bra so tight that it makes them burst out of the cleavage. The result is that they bulge out over the sides and the back as well. And a bra that's too tight leaves deep marks on the skin when you take it off, which do nothing to enhance the beauty of your breasts.

'Sometimes the familiarity of living together can lower standards of personal presentation,' she continued. 'The tradition of romantic love requires that you always cherish your body and your personal appearance. Caring for yourself will inspire your lover to value and care for you too. So treat yourself to underwear that makes you feel beautiful. Lovely satins in vibrant colours, delicate silks sewn with little pearls or sequins, a hint of lace, a tiny bow or ribbon, embroidery ... Gorgeous lingerie adds a dimension of luxury to erotic love; let it be your gift to Adam to dress for undressing, as you did when you first met.'

Padmini turned to Adam. 'There is an art to undressing your lover. The principle is to move slowly forward, while allowing delicious distractions to interrupt you. Appreciate the different textures of the clothes Eve is wearing, feel how smooth or silky they are under your hand, and feel the warmth of her body through them. Begin to unbutton, but then let your hand be diverted by the swell of her breast or the curve of her hip. Slip a finger underneath a strap and gradually tease it over her shoulder as you kiss her neck. Pay more attention to the shoulder than to the strap. The more refinements you devise for raising the erotic temperature like this, the better. When Eve thinks you're ready to move on, go back to where you were before and leave suspense to build up all on its own. Caress her shoulders, lift her hair with both hands, kiss her nape.'

'Once Eve's breasts are naked, cup them in your hands and lift them towards you so you can admire them,' suggested Koriko. 'Feel their weight and give her gentle support and uplift. She will like you looking at them like this – it's such a flattering angle. Push them up and together to create a cleavage that you can kiss. Or sit behind her and get her to lean against you, then put your arms around her so you can lift and caress her breasts from the back. This is a lovely position as she can neither see you nor reach you – all she has to do is give in to sensation and relax.'

'Feel every contour and think in to the inner woman, to her living warmth, her beating heart and the vibrant mesh of her emotions,' said Marguerite. 'Linger and appreciate every moment. Cup the side of the breast in your hand then let it fall slowly back as you pull your palm up over the curve of the breast to the centre of her chest. Move your hand in a broad circle as if you were rubbing in cream. Gentle squeezing and releasing of the whole breast with your whole hand feels wonderful. Let your touch be warm and comforting.'

'What about her nipples?' asked Adam.

'The nipples often harden with excitement like the spikes of the hyacinth,' said Padmini. 'One nipple is perhaps quicker to react than the other. Sometimes they become too tender to touch. Enjoy the signs of her arousal – they are particular to her alone, a secret waiting to be discovered. Proceed gently – breasts can be extraordinarily tender at different phases of the month. Watch to see whether the areola – the dark disc around the nipple – swells or darkens with desire. Sometimes the whole breast enlarges as blood flows into it and the delicate blue veins on the surface show more clearly. Sometimes a flush of excitement spreads across the chest. It rises from the upper belly to the tops of the breasts, then across the sides and down underneath them like a fountain. But we were talking about the nipple. A sensitive nipple can erect when a woman so much as smells her lover's scent as he walks towards her.'

'Leave close attention to the nipples till later,' said Padmini. 'For now, just brush them very lightly with the palm of your hand, and don't touch with the fingers at all. Reserve intimate contact with them for the tongue. Sweep her body with your palms, lightly stroking her flesh from the knees, up the thighs, across the breasts and down the arms to the legs again. The whole of the skin is one delicious erogenous zone. So give this serpentine caress a few times, taking in the curves of her hip and shoulder, before you narrow the circle to concentrate on her breasts. With your hands flat on the ribcage below them, push the breasts upwards between the open "V" of your thumb and the rest of your hand, but just skim the nipple very lightly with your palm as it crosses them, paying it no special attention. You can carry on like this for quite a while, varying the angle and the route of the caress – Eve will adore it.'

'Exactly how gentle and light should my touch be?' asked Adam.

'A good question,' said Koriko. 'A feather–light

touch can be ticklish and annoying and make a woman long to be held with warmth and con-fidence. Make your hand sensitive so that through your touch you gauge how firmly she would like to be held. Increase the pressure with your palm, squeeze, but not with your fingers, and make sure all your movements have a rounded quality to them, that they are sensuous and rolling and never abrupt.'

'The first time my lover ever touched my nipples', said Marguerite, 'it happened like this. He had been caressing my body all over, and homing in on my breasts with his hands so strong and delicate until I was highly aroused. Then he took his hands off my body and leaned over me. My eyes were closed in a swoon. I felt him touch my nipple with the tip of his tongue. It was the only contact between us – such an exquisite sensation, it ran right down my belly to the valley of my sex. He pressed down with his tongue quite firmly for a second or two, then started to flick the tip of the nipple lightly and rapidly with the very tip of his tongue ... I almost fainted away.'

Padmini smiled. 'One of my lovers had a technique I adored. We used to lounge on cushions in the courtyard of my house, a delightful secluded courtyard where fountains played, roses bloomed and all manner of other flowers wafted their scent about, and my peacock, Raja, strutted before us shaking out his shimmering tail feathers. My lover – he was a government minister with a harem of a hundred wives at least – would start with the tip of his tongue in the dip of my navel. Not on the button itself, you understand, which is far too sensitive for me – but on the edge of the hollow above it, which I have pierced with a ruby, as you see. Then he ran his tongue all the way up the midline of my chest, spreading it out as flat as it would go, and from there he nuzzled my breasts, clasping them to his face. He sucked the flesh of my breasts for a long, long time before he touched my nipples. He became quite abandoned, rolling his face against my breasts and sighing and sucking like a baby. Then I could bear it no longer and guided his mouth to the nipple. Well, this was such heaven. I cradled his head in my arms and he seemed to gulp and drink and suck – he made plenty of saliva – but I would swear that milk spurted from my breasts.'

'In the Orient we believe that drinking from the breasts of the beloved promotes health and long life,' said Koriko. 'We have already introduced you to the first elixir of a woman's body, the fountain of nectar that springs from her mouth. The second elixir springs from the twin fountains of her breasts. We say the essence of the nipples, which we call Heavenly Snow, is sweet tasting and has the most superior quality of all three libations, especially when drunk from a woman who has never produced milk.'

'Well!' said Padmini. 'So it's possible for the breasts to produce milk when a lover suckles there?'

'Sometimes,' said Koriko. 'And in China there are

herbal concoctions that can even produce milk in a virgin. But it doesn't matter whether the nipples secrete or not – it's the action of sucking and licking that's important. That's why we call this elixir the *essence* of the nipples, Heavenly Snow.'

'Should I nibble the nipple?' Adam wanted to know.

Marguerite smiled. 'Nibble the nipple with your closed lips if you like, but not with your teeth. Try licking the breast lavishly, as you would an ice-cream, pressing your tongue down quite hard, but when you get to the nipple, barely flick it as you pass, almost as if you had forgotten it was there. In this way you tantalize the nipple and it will ache for your touch. Then you can take it inside your mouth, and if you wish to hold it firmly, grip the bosom around it with your lips covering your teeth, and tease the tip of the nipple with your tongue. While you're sucking the nipple and it's well lubricated, you could insert your finger into your mouth and play with it as well, so Eve doesn't know where the sensation is coming from, your tongue or your finger. But whatever you do, build up slowly and always leave her wanting more – if you go too far, too fast you will break her erotic trance.'

'My lover the government minister was obsessed with my breasts,' said Padmini. 'He used to tease them with a peacock feather, or sometimes he warmed his mouth with a hot drink before he fastened it to my nipple, or cooled it with a cold one. He used to blindfold me and subject me to all the sensations of his fantasy. He would pucker his lips onto my nipple and make a "vvv–vvv" sound, vibrating energy and warmth through my breast. One of his favourite delights was to smear my breasts with honey or cream, then slowly lick it all off.'

Marguerite bent forward and whispered to Eve: 'Adam will find it very arousing to watch you caress your breasts. Cup them in your hands and offer them to him like a goddess, then give him a massage with your nipples. Lean over him as he lies back on the bed and rub them gently across his naked body.'

Eve instinctively pressed her hands to her heart chakra as she dreamed of the sensual delights that were to come.

SCROLL 5

The Unfolding Lotus

❧

The Courtesans' Parchment

The sacred lotus of the East is a plant of unique loveliness. It is said to be the first of all flowers, because it rises in perfect beauty out of stagnant water.

N THE WEST, FEMALE SEXUALITY HAS traditionally been seen as passive, but in the East it is the energizing force of the universe. In ancient India and China the female sex organs were regarded with awe as the seat of human power and the wellspring of all creativity. This reverence is expressed in the world's oldest name for the female genitals, the Sanskrit word yoni, which means 'sacred place'. The earliest sign of the *yoni* – an upright oval with pointed ends – reflects the shape of the vulva when aroused and swollen. The ancients loved to depict the yoni in its excited state and celebrated it as a paradise island they called Jambu, in the heart of which was *vajrasana*, the clitoris, the Diamond Seat of the Seventh Heaven.

The most complex and potent of the many symbols of the yoni that the ancients found in the natural world was the lotus. The sacred lotus of the East is a plant of unique loveliness. It is said to be the first of all flowers, because it rises in perfect beauty out of stagnant water. Its film–coated leaves collect glittering droplets of dew, which settle on them like jewels. The flower stalk bears three large egg–shaped buds that open one after the other into heavenly–scented translucent white or pink blossoms the size of a halo. A double lotus has more than fifty succulent petals delicately suffused with colour, reminiscent of the complex unfolding anatomy of the yoni.

Rising out of murky darkness to flower in radiant sunlight, the lotus is the mystic flower of enlightenment. For Buddhists and Hindus it reflects the spiritual purity of the soul as it flies free from the turbulent waters of worldly striving, attachment and desire. To sit in the lotus position, with the legs folded into the trunk of the body like petals, and the chin tucked in so that the eyes gaze directly forwards, effortlessly lengthens and straightens the spine. The vertebrae seem to float free of one another and to hang from heaven like a golden thread or a string of pearls. The alignment of the spine opens the pathway of the spinal cord, connecting the body's nervous system directly to the energy of the heavens. To form a circuit of psychic energy with their arms as well as their legs, seekers rested the backs of their hands on their knees and pressed the pads of their thumbs and index fingers together in the *yoni mudra*, the sign of the vulva. The same yonic finger sign is used by people who practise meditation in the West today, though many may be unaware of its meaning.

Contemplating their energetic connection to the heavens while sitting in the lotus position, the ancients discovered that there were seven whirling vortices of energy strung like jewels along the spine, which they called *chakras*, the Sanskrit word for wheel.

❦ The first or root chakra lies at the base of the spine;

❦ the second, sacral chakra, is midway between the pubic bone and the navel;

❦ the third, solar plexus chakra, lies above the navel and between the ribs;

❦ the fourth, heart chakra, between the breasts;

❦ the fifth, throat chakra, at the Adam's apple;

❦ the sixth, third eye chakra, between the eyebrows;

❦ and the seventh, crown chakra, at the top of the head.

These sites of extraordinary energetic activity recognized by the ancients correspond in the physical
body to densely bundled plexuses of nerves.
Furthermore, as was discovered only in the
twentieth century, their positions reflect almost
exactly the site of the endocrine glands, whose
major function is to secrete the hormones that
govern the body's sexuality.

As they meditated, the ancients visualized each
highly charged chakra as a perfect lotus with a
different number of petals. They found that the
energy of each chakra vibrated at its own frequency
and that they could reproduce this frequency in
sound by uttering words of power they called a
mantra, meaning 'to think' and 'to release'. The
mantra invoked the energy of the chakra, a
heavenly vibration with its own individual qualities
that resonate in human experience. To think of the
heavenly or the divine and then to let go of all
thought was the object of meditation, for this in
turn released divine energy. The energy of each

chakra also resonated with a particular scent, colour and symbol, all of which provided more sensual aids to meditation.

The path of enlightenment starts at Muladhara, the root chakra. This is the seat of physicality where the slumbering life force of the coiled serpent Kundalini resides. Through meditation on each of the seven chakras in turn, the seeker feels the serpent of energy uncoil and rise right up the spine to the crown, where it flowers in an emanation of spiritual light – just as the lotus grows in mud and blooms in heavenly splendour. Thus spiritual enlightenment arises out of contemplating earthy physicality in relaxation and openness – the sexual and the spiritual become one. The cycle is ever-lasting – from flower to seed, from decay to regeneration as the Kundalini serpent rises and falls in a spiral around the spine.

To the Tantrics, who followed the path of erotic mysticism, enlightenment came not just from sitting still in meditation, but also from actively celebrating the sacred within the profane. They reached enlightenment through intimate knowledge of female sexual power, exploring all aspects of the yoni and all parts of the lotus, from its rhizomes growing in the mud to its glorious petals alive with light.

The Tantrics discovered that the lotus not only looks like the yoni but, like the intense sexual experience of the yoni, has the power to alter the perceptions, filling the mind and spirit with soaring elation. It is one of a small group of plants called plants of immortality or entheogenic plants, which are said to induce experiences of the divine. When the lotus is properly prepared, drinking the resultant juice can produce a luminous mystical experience with visionary lights and supernatural sounds and a feeling of radiant joy and inspiration. The Tantrics made the lotus into a drink they called *soma*, which they drank in celebration of the earthly and spiritual power of sex. When the soma of the lotus was drunk by those in love, it was said to induce an ecstasy that brought expansion beyond this life, a perception of awesome vastness surpassing both heaven and earth. The chemical composition of the lotus has an effect very like that of a drug synthetically manufactured in the modern age, 3,4-methylene-dioxymethamphetamine (MDMA), popularly known as Ecstasy.

Though the soma drink of the lotus was taken to intensify erotic love, the goal of the mystic was to reach ecstasy by liberating the body and mind in new realms of erotic experience without either drugs or superficial visual stimulation. Because the lotus bears bud, blossom and seed pod together, it spoke to the ancients of the triple goddess who shows all three aspects of woman: virgin, mother and crone. A Tantric worshipper seeking union with the goddess might be met at the temple door by her priestess in the guise of a wizened old woman. Unless he could adore the sublime goddess alive inside her with both his body and his mind, he would not be admitted to the inner sanctum. But if the priestess appeared at the threshold of the temple as a ravishing beauty, he was to use all his willpower to resist her erotic charms. Instead he had to meditate on her loveliness until he could also experience her old age and even beyond that, her death and the decomposition of her corpse. Only when he could embrace all earthly aspects of womankind in this one woman would his sexual experience be spiritually complete. It was a lesson in reaching the divine, the ultimate erotic bliss, through total acceptance of the most basic realities of life, and it involved the most difficult emotional adjustment of rejecting all personal prejudices and attachments. It was also a lesson in taking complete responsibility for one's own sexual fulfilment, and in liberating oneself from the crutches of blaming circumstances or the beloved for the lack of it.

All over the East the lotus was the emblem of female sexuality not only as a creative force, but also as destroyer. The yoni was the gateway of life and death, a gateway seen everywhere in the Hindu and Arab worlds in the familiar horseshoe archway of traditional architecture. This archway made the comings and goings of all who passed through it take on a deeper symbolic dimension. It inspired the European custom of nailing a horseshoe to the door and the Western practice of giving the bride a lucky silver horseshoe to carry on her wedding day. Of course the horseshoe should have its feet pointing earthwards to fulfil its true function as a fertility charm.

The horseshoe arch forms omega, the last letter of the Greek alphabet. 'The Alpha and the Omega', the beginning and the end, was originally the mantra of the great goddess who ruled life's entrance and exit. The words of the Egyptian supreme goddess Saïs were carved in stone on her temple: 'I am all that has been, that is, and that will be.' In Egypt the blue lotus that floats dreamily on the waters of the Nile was Saïs, the mother of all creation, the goddess of the feminine elements earth and water from whose body the male sun rose at the birth of the universe.

But Saïs also devoured the sun when it set. The creative and destructive female forces combined most potently in the archetypal Indian goddess of the lotus, Kali. With her terrifying bloody fangs, her staring eyes and her red yoni full of snakes, Kali was the tomb as well as the womb, the Dark Mother who squatted over the body of her dead consort Shiva while her yoni swallowed up his lingam. She was the ancients' awe and terror of female sexuality, their belief that its power could snatch away the life of the lingam and the life of man as well as give them life. Tantric worshippers of Kali had to endure their dread of her curse before they could fully experience the joy of her blessing.

In biblical times in the Middle East the all-powerful lotus goddess was usurped by a male deity, who took on her triple aspect in the form of the Father, the Son and the Holy Ghost. A thousand years after it was inscribed on her Egyptian temple, he also adopted her mantra 'the Alpha and the Omega' as his title of omnipotence. Early versions of the Bible's Genesis story robbed woman of her creative role and made her sexuality manageable by cutting her personality into two. According to Hebrew tradition, Adam's first wife was Lilith, named after *lilu*, the lily, otherwise known as the blue lotus of the Nile. Lilith refused to lie beneath Adam to have intercourse with him, because it brought her no satisfaction. So she left her sexually unawakened husband to his ignorance and crossed the desert to the Red Sea, which is named for the churning sea of her menstrual blood. And there by its deep salty waters she cavorted with demons and found at last the ecstasy she was seeking. Meanwhile, the unimaginative Adam had married again. But though Eve presented God with the more acceptable face of womankind, He still blamed her for arousing erotic thoughts in her husband. She offered Adam the fruit of her sexual wisdom, the apple from the forbidden tree, and in His anger at Adam's erection God made the pair cover their genitals, which were henceforth known as pudenda, meaning 'shameful'. And to punish Eve for the balmy erotic interlude in the paradise garden, He made her responsible for the curse of Original Sin, which He decreed should be passed down through generations immemorial.

The Church authorities of medieval Europe so feared the power of female sexuality that they denounced the lotus position because of its sexual connotations – and even accused people who sat cross-legged of sorcery. But the cult of Courtly Love that flowered in the early Middle Ages secretly pursued the Eastern adoration of woman and celebrated her erotic power in epic stories of knights who quested after the Holy Grail. The mysterious Grail was variously described as a chalice, a womb, a symbol of rebirth, a vessel filled with holy blood, a dispenser of joy, a cauldron supplying never-ending sustenance, a horn of plenty; it was none other than the mystic lotus blossom, the eternal yoni.

The symbol of the yoni filtered irresistibly into

mainstream Western culture, and eventually the oval with pointed ends was adopted by the Church as its own emblem – but set on its side and called a fish. However, stonemasons who worked on medieval churches knew the true meaning of the symbol and respected its power. Scattered across Europe are churches that feature grotesque stone carvings of women squatting and holding their yonis open with their fingers for all to see – in Ireland these figures are known as Sheila–na–gigs. They are similar to the carvings of women exposing their yonis that can be seen decorating temple doorways in India, where tradition holds that everyone who enters touches the sacred yoni to bless themselves.

The Conversation

Feel the energy building inside,

radiating out to enliven your skin

then spreading way beyond you

into the world.

ADAM AND EVE AND THE THREE courtesans were carried up the mountainside in a colourful procession of sedan chairs. Eventually they emerged on to a broad plateau and the bearers set the quaint conveyances gently on the ground. The landscape could have come straight out of a Taoist painting. In the distance, lofty, needle–shaped mountains lost their heads in the cloud; far below a yellow ribbon of river snaked its way through a wide valley. All around were huge boulders and crags of granite to which gnarled trees and shrubs clung with marvellous tenacity. The awesome scale of the scene and the purity of the mountain air made all their senses come alive.

'This is the shrine of the goddess,' said Koriko, pointing to a fissure in a thickly wooded cliff. 'Many ancient shrines to the goddess were yonic clefts in a rock hidden under tangled vegetation, or caves overgrown with the tendrils of vines secluded deep in a forest or grove.'

'Eastern reverence for the power of the yoni embraced even the mat of dense curly hair that protects the female pubis,' said Padmini. 'In India both mystics and gypsies used the sacred triangle to communicate with the divine – mystics meditated upon the shape, while the gypsies laid out their Tarot cards in a triangle for divination.'

'In dreams and the mythic imagination,' said Marguerite, 'female pubic hair has a disturbing part to play, for it conceals the buried treasure of sexual delight and frustrates the seeker near his goal. The impenetrable forest has a symbolic significance in any quest, for to get lost in it is to immerse oneself in the dark world of the unconscious, the wilderness through which one must pass before reaching enlightenment. Being lost in the forest means not that one must be found, but that one must find oneself. In Tantra, this life–changing journey is the path to wisdom and sexual awakening.'

'The fifth step on your way to the Seventh Heaven is a momentous one,' said Koriko, inviting them all to sit with her in front of the rocky shrine, 'for it gives intimate knowledge of the lotus. We are here today to immerse ourselves, as the ancients did before us, in a sensual exploration of woman's sacred place.'

'For you, Eve, this means understanding and intensifying your orgasmic power and the power of your sexuality,' said Padmini. 'And for you, Adam, it means discovering an exquisite variety of erotic pleasures for Eve, so that you can increase your sexual power and be blessed and strengthened in her love.'

'We will begin by imagining the female form

naked,' said Marguerite. 'And as the goddess turns towards us we will gaze in rapture and without shame upon her loveliness.'

'To men throughout the ancient world a smooth and hairless female body represented beauty, youth, innocence – and accessibility,' said Padmini. 'So women have always been eager to remove the hair that grows in such wild abundance on their pubis, and along with it a symbolic barrier to their sexuality. Indian women pulled out their pubic hairs with an arrangement of threads like a cat's cradle, which they manipulated between their fingers. The Egyptians invented herbal depilatory creams and developed the technique of "sugaring" with a sticky emulsion made of oil and honey. The Greeks used tweezers, or singed off the hairs with a burning lamp; sometimes they rubbed at them with hot ashes. In Rome they devised a way of "waxing" unwanted body hair with resin or pitch. And these painful processes repaid the effort, for they revealed the smooth fleshy mound of the mons Veneris, the mount of Venus, the soft pad of fat named after the goddess of love that covers the pubic bone and fits snugly inside a man's cupped hand.'

'The mount of Venus is highly sensitive to being held and caressed,' said Koriko, 'because, as your modern scientists tell us, it is richly endowed with super-sensory nerve endings not usually found in hairy skin. When the fleshy mound is stroked, chemical changes take place in the nerve endings at the hair follicles, which combine with the reactions of nerve endings in the skin to increase sexual excitement. Experiment, Adam, and you will see that simply rubbing, squeezing and rocking the mons in the warmth of your hand creates delicious indirect pressure on the clitoris. So erotic is the feeling induced there that it can bring some women to orgasm, especially when combined with caressing the breasts and deep, prolonged kissing.'

'To continue our exploration of the goddess,' said Marguerite to Adam, 'imagine sliding your hand down her mount of Venus towards her thighs and pushing them gently apart. You will see there two folds of flesh, the labia majora or outer lips, which meet at a central cleft, like the one in this shrine before us. This cleft is called the *rima*. It opens in sexual excitement as the lips swell and part to reveal the coral grotto of the vulva or yoni, woman's sacred place. It is one of life's great gifts for every man to study and appreciate the secret geography of the yoni and to realize that in both appearance and response, the yoni of his beloved is unique and subtly different from that of all other women.

'So I urge you to gaze on the yoni of your beloved; look at the detail of the treasures it holds for you. Notice how the outer lips, when swollen with desire, are smooth, slick and dark pink or red, like the ripe fruit of the fig. These lips cradle a smaller plump pair of ruby-red lips, the labia minora ...'

Koriko let out a deep sigh. 'The English sexual vocabulary jars on my ears. It is either too clinical and cold or too crude for tender use in the bed-room. Our Oriental terminology is just the opposite – colourful and poetic, full of reverence for the sexual parts of a woman in its allusions to precious gems and the wonders of nature. Besides being romantic and picturesque, our language gives a much more specific geography of the yoni and opens the way towards a more sensuously detailed knowledge of lovemaking. I recommend you try it.

'What you so formally call the labia minora, we call the Red Petals, because of their glowing, translucent beauty. Between them, the deep dark red opening of the vagina is the Cinnabar Cave, a vivid and appropriate name because cinnabar is a precious red mineral with aphrodisiac qualities found where there are volcanoes and hot springs. The Golden Spring, the opening of the urethra, lies just above it. Its name tells its function. And at the top of the yonic oval is the clitoris, called the Diamond Seat of the Seventh Heaven.

'The Diamond is the only part of any living being

that exists solely to give pleasure. It contains twice as many nerve endings as the man has in his Jade Stalk. Understandably, such a highly sensitive organ cannot always bear direct touch. The Diamond withdraws by sliding smoothly under a tent formed by the tips of the Red Petals as they join above it. We call this exquisitely sensitive tent the Heavenly Wings.

'The Diamond is dark pink, moist and shiny, and if you look closely, you will see that it has a wrinkled "collar" that corresponds exactly to the wrinkled skin beneath the head of the Jade Stalk. While you call this the frenulum, our poetic name for it is the Lute Strings, because of the erotic delight they give, like celestial music, when gently stroked.

'We have two other names for which you have no translation. The Golden Gulley is the deliciously tender upper part of the yoni and the Jade Vein is the lower part. Each has its own vibration of sexual feeling and a woman will sometimes prefer the upper one to be stimulated, and at other times, the lower. All of these names will be very useful for you, Eve, in giving precise instructions to Adam. Working delicately with his fingers, he will be able to refine his technique of stimulating your yoni to give you the most varied and intense pleasure.'

'Practise the art of communication during your lovemaking,' Marguerite urged them. 'As you lovingly touch Eve's yoni, be aware of the detail of sexual geography under your fingers. Ask her to describe how it feels and say what she would like you to try next. Using the vocabulary we have given you, conduct your own erotic exploration.'

'The arousal of the yoni is fascinating to watch,' said Padmini. 'As Eve's excitement grows under your touch, you will see her clitoris and its shaft darken as they fill with blood and erect just like your penis does. But what many lovers don't realize, because it is never taught in your modern world, is that the clitoris is just the tip of the female erection, which is comparable in size to that of the male.

'The only difference between your erection and Eve's is that hers is internal. But still you can witness dramatic changes by studying her yoni. As the clitoris erects, it can double in size and push out shiny and dark from under its tent. The labia redden and swell until they stand thrust open by their own voluptuous excitement as blood rushes in, engorging the tissue. Glands secrete salty–sweet lubricating juices. Eve may be awash with secretions, or she may barely get slippery, or be wet one moment and dry the next; natural juices dry very quickly.'

'As Eve's sexual tension increases,' said Marguerite, 'her clitoris may become so sensitive that it disappears again to protect itself from direct stimulation.'

'Her breathing becomes faster and shallower,' said Padmini. 'Her blood pressure and pulse rate reach a peak as she moves towards orgasm; and suddenly she feels a sensation of swelling, tightening, lifting, rushing, followed by release in the form of exquisite rhythmic pulsing.'

'There may be many spasms or few,' said Marguerite; 'gradually they become less intense and less frequent. Orgasm causes contractions of the pelvic floor muscles in both men and women, and they even pulse at the same rhythm – one contraction every four–fifths of a second.'

'Learn to anticipate Eve's orgasm and study the reactions of her body,' suggested Koriko. 'Every woman behaves differently and sometimes it takes close observation to recognize what is happening. Because while some writhe and thrash uncontrollably, others tense and retreat inwards, lying rigid and still. The legs may stiffen, the back arch, the teeth grit; all the muscles can tense and the feet point outwards. The body may convulse; she may moan and grip hold of you, her eyes rolling, her head thrown back. Japanese erotic art offers acute observations of women in orgasm; it depicts them with faces frozen and toes violently curled.'

'After orgasm,' said Marguerite, 'a woman returns to the pre–orgasmic state, and not, like a man, to the pre-sexual state. In this phase she may feel over-whelming tenderness that verges on tears, and a desire to hold her beloved close. Deep relaxation coexists with the sense of being charged with energy, health and vitality; mind and thought are positively absent. The release from mental process-ing, worry and pain; the absolute glow of love, warmth and generosity; the awareness of physical bliss – this is the state of enlightenment that mystics have always striven for, and which the ancients knew that woman alone possessed.'

'The ancients also knew that from this plateau of bliss a woman could rise again to experience orgasm after orgasm', said Padmini. 'This is because – unlike in the male – each contraction that squeezes blood from the erectile tissues is followed immediately by a vacuum that is refilled; distension creates more engorgement and swelling, which leads to more tension and the possibility of further orgasm, or slow subsidence back to the pre-sexual state. Because the female erectile tissues are internal and not external, as in a man, the blood supply to them is inexhaustible. This was what the ancients meant by "the inexhaustible female". The gypsies knew it too. Their king traditionally employed a man called a "tickler" to keep his queen satisfied, and to prepare her for sex with him.'

'Although many women may not realize it,' said Koriko to Eve, 'whether to have one orgasm or several is a matter of personal choice for each of us. The Oriental name for orgasm is Yin Tide, which speaks of a phenomenon that naturally recurs. I know a famous Japanese erotic print that shows a courtesan quietly enjoying her thirty-third orgasm of the night; only her curled toes betray her inner emotion. The Taoists believed that a man was strengthened by his lover's orgasm; the more climaxes he gave her, the longer he would live. However, it is the quality of the experience and not the number of orgasms that counts: many climaxes are not better than one. To some women, the clitoris feels too sensitive to touch – even indirectly through the mons – after one orgasm. More stimulation too soon could also diffuse and dull the feeling and make another orgasm impossible. A sensitive lover will let his partner take the lead and accept her wishes either way.'

'I am confused about the role the vagina plays in female orgasm,' said Adam. 'Or perhaps it plays no role at all?'

'I can understand your confusion,' said Koriko, 'because only in the last century did your scientists discover what we in the East have known for thousands of years, namely that the clitoris and not the vagina is the seat of sexual response. Even today most of your textbooks do not feature the full female erectile system and your sex education books for children are particularly responsible for perpetuating ignorance about female sexuality. They discuss the penis, erection and ejaculation, but ignore the clitoris and female sexual response altogether – their excuse being that these are not necessary for reproduction.'

'The word vagina means "sheath" or "scabbard", which shows its function from the male point of view', said Padmini. 'The vagina is important in sex mainly as a receptacle for a penis. The *Kamasutra* defines women by the size of their vagina, dividing them into Deer, Mares and Elephants, corresponding to the male penis sizes of Hare, Bull and Stallion. In reality the size of the vagina varies little, being slightly larger in a woman who has given birth. While the grip of the vagina around the penis regularly brings men to orgasm, vaginal penetration does not perform the same favour for most women. This is of course because the true seat of pleasure, the clitoris, gets little or no stimulation during penetrative sex. On your journey to the Seventh Heaven you are discovering how to intensify erotic pleasure. This is the reason why you have – for the time being – given up penetration, with all its potential for disappointments and anxieties, and its unreliability in giving women orgasm.'

'However,' said Marguerite, 'Western science has supplied us with some useful information about the sensitivity of the vagina. The outer third of the vagina contains nearly ninety per cent of vaginal nerve endings, which are highly concentrated around the vaginal opening in the vulva. The less sensitive inner two–thirds still respond to firmer stimulation.'

'So paying attention to the Cinnabar Cave, our poetic name for the vaginal opening, will be well rewarded,' said Koriko with a smile. 'It is indeed a deliciously sensitive spot. And it feels the full force of the contractions of orgasm as they grip the muscles of the pelvic floor.'

'I expect you know that in a virgin, the vaginal opening is sometimes covered by a membrane called the hymen or maidenhead,' said Marguerite. 'Hymen was the Greek god of marriage and his name means "veil". The rupturing of the hymen as the virgin is deflowered is symbolically enacted when the bride lifts her veil to receive the groom's kiss. I tell you this, Eve, for though you have given up intercourse for a while, the idea of *the veiled erotic* is a potent one in the male imagination. When a man glimpses a secret curve of his lover's body through fragile lace, delicate gauze or filmy silk, it fires his imagination and acts as a seductive challenge. And now you know the origin of this male impulse!

'So I suggest you wear a loose silk wrap while Adam studies the secret places of your yoni,' she whispered to Eve. 'And perhaps lacy French knickers or culottes. Tell him that he can look but not touch as you pull the lace aside and open the petals of your lotus flower to expose your yoni. The chances are that you will find being the object of his erotic study very arousing, even though you may feel a little shy at first, and what could be more natural than to want to heighten your arousal and his desire by pleasuring yourself? You can do this slowly and gently, naming the places that you love to touch, while Adam continues to watch without touching you, however much he wants to.'

'The way you put it makes it sound so lovely,' said Eve.

Marguerite smiled. 'It is simply the most natural way to discover your body's sexual response and learn about the changes it goes through on the way to orgasm. It is a comforting way of loving and caring for oneself.'

'Make yourself a luxurious nest among pillows and cushions,' said Padmini, 'and for Adam's sake wear a little jewellery with your lace. I like to sit or lie with my legs spread, lifting my heels and pulling up my knees. This stretches the yoni, intensifying sensations and offering your lover a perfect view. When I am alone sometimes I lie on my stomach, so that I can press and thrust my mons against the couch and squeeze my thighs together rhythmically to stimulate my Diamond indirectly. In the bath, a tingling water massage with the jets from a shower hose can create a delicious stimulation that is at once specific and diffuse. Some women like to dip a fingertip just inside the Cinnabar Cave as they stimulate the Diamond, while others find it a distraction.'

'Creating time in which to caress oneself to orgasm is a heavenly experience that lifts the mood and energizes mind and body,' said Koriko. 'Every woman needs it, whether she does it herself, or relaxes to her lover's touch. Rhythmic stimulation creates a warm and spreading glow that gradually builds up with electric feelings of intense, irresistible sensitivity to a trance-like, urgent draw. Then a tremendous surge of tension is followed by a trembling and a swooning, and the climax breaks like a tidal wave, radiating outwards from the Diamond through the yoni as the whole body arches and relaxes. All sense of time is lost in enveloping bliss.'

❧

Eve wondered if the courtesans would ever recommend the use of a dildo.

'Your fingers are warm, sensitive, alive to your needs', said Marguerite. 'Dildoes are just things. And as we have told you, penetration does not stimulate the clitoris and there are relatively few sensitive nerve endings inside the vagina. However, women have used dildoes since prehistoric times, and if you like the idea, you can by all means use one, well oiled, to stimulate the delicate parts of your yoni.'

'In ancient India dildoes were made of precious materials', said Padmini: 'gold, silver and ivory; and sometimes they were made of wood, tin or even lead! For solitary pleasure or for mutual use in the harem, we used bulbous gourds or roots, well oiled, or bundles of reeds tied together and softened with the extracts of plants.'

'In Japan the dildo, which we call *harigata*, was a popular feature in erotic prints of beautiful geishas or nuns', said Koriko. '*Harigata* were works of art, carved in wood or finely moulded in hand–painted porcelain. Some represented the mythical Otafuku, patron of feminine sexual appetite, or the erotic goddess Benten; others were phallic replicas, pro-duced in painstaking detail and with ferociously swollen veins. In Japanese erotic art the phallus is traditionally massive, way out of proportion to the rest of the male body. *Harigata* were enormous too. Some were made of leather, buffalo horn or tortoiseshell and soaked in warm water before use to give the correct blend of firmness and flexibility. Some models were fixed to the heel – so convenient in a country where kneeling was the common position for relaxation!

'And then we had *rin-no-tama*, "bell balls", little erotic toys designed to be slipped into the vagina, the Hidden Place, and worn while not engaged in sex to bring an erotic *frisson* to everyday life. The Japanese believed these balls originated in China during the Ming dynasty and contained drops of saliva from a mythical bird. This was thought to be such a potent aphrodisiac that it would boil when the balls were warmed in the hand, causing the bells inside them to ring.

'Modern Japanese *rin-no-tama* are hardly different from what they were in the fifteenth century – a pair of silver balls, one containing a blob of mercury and the other a tongue of copper. The balls do indeed vibrate when held on the palm of the hand and they may act like a tuning fork to emit a high–pitched sound. Some women claim they produce a whole range of exquisite sensations by knocking against one another inside the Hidden Place as they move.'

*

'So now we explore the path to a more powerful orgasm,' said Padmini, turning to Eve. 'Let me encourage you to be more aware of your latent eroticism in everyday life. You can express this in the ways you dress, move and interact with people, but its essence is a subtle glow of inner sexual confidence that will be unmistakable in its allure to the opposite sex. Daily exercises in sexual awareness will develop both confidence and orgasmic potential.

'My favourite way of releasing sexual energy is to move the pelvis, letting it circle freely around the centre of the body. From ancient times, the sensuous art of belly dancing has been known for its power to heal and strengthen sexual experience, as well as for its mesmerizing erotic effect on the men who watch it. So practise this dance for Adam.

'Stand freely, feeling yourself centred in your belly. Drop your shoulders. Focus your mind on the dot of your navel. An awareness of the belly as the centre of the self gives solidity and stability; it opens the way to sexual confidence.

'Put your hands on your hips and imagine the life force of the Kundalini serpent coiled inside your pelvis. Let your pelvis begin to move in very small circles as the serpent uncurls. The circles grow slowly wider, becoming more daring as your power spreads out from your navel through your belly. Push to the right, thrust your pelvis provocatively forward and roll your hips over to the left. Push to the rear. Keep your torso upright! The more you practise, the smoother the circle will get as tension in the hips is released. Feel the energy building inside, radiating out to enliven your skin then spreading way beyond you into the world. Roll your hips in a big circle as if you were swinging the moon in its orbit round your waist. Let your energy stream out towards the stars.'

Eve got up to join in and the two women lost themselves in the gyrating rhythm of the dance.

'And now another exercise', said Padmini. 'The belly wave. It imitates the contractions of labour and puts you in direct contact with your sexuality. The belly wave exercises the muscles of the pelvic floor, strengthening the contractions of orgasm – and is often recommended after childbirth.

'Begin by placing both thumbs on your navel with your palms flat on your lower belly. Imagine your ovaries beneath your palms. Thrust the lower belly out, then pull it in and up as far as you can, pulling up your diaphragm too. Now push your diaphragm out and let your belly roll down and out. Begin slowly, then as you repeat the sequence, you can speed up and maintain a smoothly pulsating rhythm. In Arabic countries women practise the belly wave to the rhythm of a drum. It is highly erotic to watch.'

Their bared bellies rolled and shuddered under their hands, fluttering and vibrating. Soon Eve was out of breath, but she could already feel the sexual pull on her pelvic floor muscles and realized how much they would benefit from daily exercise.

'A five-minute session of belly dancing every day will strengthen those muscles in just a week or two,' Padmini promised her.

'The pelvic floor muscles involved in orgasm are centred on the perineum,' said Koriko. 'That's the muscular bridge between the genitals and the anus. In the Orient we call it the Gate of Life and Death. It's central to all Eastern spiritual and sexual practices, but so neglected in the West that many people don't even know its name.'

Padmini agreed. 'In India the perineum

represents the strength of the whole body. When a baby is born, anyone assisting at the labour will continually massage the mother's perineum to draw her awareness into it and allow it to work with her, making it much less likely to tear as the baby's head emerges.'

'Daily exercises that involve the muscles of the perineum will be most effective for improving the power of your orgasm,' said Koriko. 'Any time you are sitting down you can exercise in private by clenching and releasing these muscles. I usually do this one hundred times twice a day. Test your strength by trying to stop a stream of urine in full flow.'

'Is there any way I can boost the power of my orgasm while it's actually happening?' asked Eve.

'Certainly,' said Koriko. 'We can recommend five simple techniques that will help you enjoy the most profound orgasms you have ever experienced. All but the first work equally well for men. But while they are simple to perform, they are difficult to remember, because they are designed for the moments just before and during orgasm when you are not used to thinking of anything. However, we urge you to try them, and in time you may be able to combine all four, and experience orgasms of tremendous power.

The first intensifies the sensitivity of the whole yoni during stimulation by fingers or tongue. Spread your legs and stroke your lower belly firmly towards your yoni. Use your palms or the heels of your hands and press down as you push, imagining the energy streaming from the ovaries beneath your hands to your clitoris.

The second is to place your tongue on the roof of your mouth as you feel the tide of orgasm seething within you. This closes an energy circuit that runs round the body from the perineum up the spine to the crown chakra at the top of the head, then down the front through the heart chakra and the navel to the perineum again. When you close the circuit orgasmic energy can course freely around it and you can feel your orgasm vibrate throughout your whole body.

The third is powerfully to pull up your perineum and tighten your anus at the same time. This is another way of closing the energy circuit and spreading orgasmic vibrations throughout the body.

The fourth technique is to pump the perineum again and again. This can trigger orgasm if you are ready, or strengthen the explosion of an orgasm that is already bursting.

The midpoint on the perineum is known by the beautiful name of Stairway to Heaven because of its role in sexual life. Pressure on this point amplifies the sensations at orgasm. So the fifth technique is to practise pressing in quite deeply with your forefinger at the first pulse of the orgasm. This is a good exercise for your lover to perform for you.'

*

Now the courtesans turned their attention to Adam. The yoni is of course more private to a woman than the Jade Stalk is to a man,' said Marguerite. 'The yoni is hidden and internal, a buried treasure, and a woman's arousal is a slow, secret process that cannot be hurried. But one of the mysteries of woman is her unpredictable and infinite variety, and her sexuality can also be overt, and passionately demanding. Whatever her sexual mood, the way to arouse her to new peaks of desire is to match your pace and timing to her needs, but always – until the very end – to hold just a little in reserve, so that her need increases in urgency. Though you may be controlling the game, let her take the lead so that she is begging you for more. And only when her feelings are fully engaged, and her skin, her mouth, her breasts, are fully aroused, should you allow yourself to touch the hot, wet, intimate place of her yoni.

'Her inner thighs are very sensitive. Warm them with the heat of your hands, brushing and caressing lightly upwards with lingering, confident caresses. If you are lying beside your love embracing and kissing her, slip your hand between her thighs and hold her yoni in your palm, pressing it closed. Press down firmly on her mount of Venus, rocking and pulling it gently. Kiss her passionately so she is desperate for you to slip a finger inside, but all the while hold back. This is the way to increase her ardour.

'Then move down her body so that you can watch her arousal. Spread her legs with your palms, and rest your head on her thigh like a pillow. Keep one hand free to caress her belly. Without touching her with your tongue, press your open lips to the skin of her upper thigh and breathe warm air onto it. Move your mouth closer to her yoni. Part the thicket of the pubic hair and delicately open the outer lips, and again without touching, gently breathe warm air onto her open yoni.'

'Begin to explore her yoni with your fingers,' said Padmini in a low voice, 'making them wet with saliva or oil. Trace its shape as if you had never seen or touched the secret parts of a woman before.

Remember all the erotic geography we have taught you and begin to pay detailed attention to each delicious feature. As the yoni engorges with blood and opens out to you like a flower, you can explore more deeply. Find the groove of the Golden Gulley; below it circle the Cinnabar Cave; below that, rub the Jade Vein. Read Eve's responses carefully and let them dictate your movements. Notice how the Diamond strains from the tent of the Heavenly Wings and play on the Wings with a feather-light touch. Whisk up light flicking, tickling or rubbing movements with your fingers and let them stray from one treasure to the next and back again. Use less pressure than you think you need so her body continually begs you for more. Gradually build up rhythm and speed as if you were playing a living musical instrument. Give her plenty of time, and plenty more. This is your gift to her. Lose yourself in the delicious art you are practising.'

'As her breathing and heartbeat begin to change,' murmured Koriko, 'she might make little thrusting movements towards you with her pelvis. Dip the very tip of your finger quickly in and out of her Cinnabar Cave; let it play fast, like a darting tongue taking nectar from a flower. Dip in a little deeper if she wants, but always keep her yearning for more by returning to flick lightly at the rim.'

'Move up the Golden Gulley to the Diamond,' said Padmini. 'See how it swells out of its Heavenly Wings. Play the Lute Strings with your finger. Keep up your rhythm and speed. As she strains towards you flick the Diamond with the tip of your middle finger, allowing your other fingers and the heel of your hand to continue to rub and tickle her yoni as you move.'

'As she reaches her climax,' whispered Koriko, 'her face and chest are flushed, her muscles go into spasm. Keep going until she convulses –' She breathed out slowly. 'And then she will need firm pressure, along the Golden Gulley and the Jade Vein; perhaps she would like a finger inserted firmly inside the Hidden Place; perhaps a whole palm over her yoni, with a fingertip pressure against the Stairway to Heaven on the perineum. You must ask her.'

Silence fell softly. Adam realized that he had been in a kind of trance. He looked from Koriko to Marguerite.

'And what should I do next?' he asked.

'Do whatever Eve wants you to do,' said Marguerite. 'Eve will be at her strongest and her most vulnerable. Accept her emotions. Hold her in your arms. Ask her if she wants more.'

'Bringing a woman to bliss with your fingers is a delicate technique,' said Padmini. 'You should take every opportunity to practise.'

'The human body has many mysteries,' said Koriko. 'Your sexuality is unique to your body and personality and only you and your lover can begin to know it and revere its secrets. You are on a journey of intimate sexual discovery. It is not necessary to measure yourself against any outside standard, only to let your sexuality unfold – like the lotus.'

SCROLL 6

The Holy Kiss

❧

The Courtesans' Parchment

Wherever it is grown and enjoyed, the fig is a reminder of the intimate details of female sexual anatomy. Hidden inside the soft outer body, the ripe fruit is blood red, moist, honey-sweet and succulent.

You held my lotus blossom
In your lips and played with the
Pistil. We took one piece of
Magic rhinoceros horn
And could not sleep all night long.
All night the cock's gorgeous crest
Stood erect. All night the bee
Clung trembling to the flower
Stamens. Oh my sweet perfumed
Jewel! I will allow only
My lord to possess my sacred
Lotus pond, and every night
You can make blossom in me
Flowers of fire.

This beautiful love song was written in the sixteenth century by Huang O, the daughter of the President of the Board of Works at China's Ming Court; she was unique in her time as a female writer of erotic verse who was not a courtesan. The words were sung to the tune *Soaring Clouds*, and anyone

who knew the melody would have a better understanding of the lovers' night of bliss. 'Clouds and
rain' was the picturesque expression for intercourse.
Clouds represented the gathering storm of female
orgasmic power; rain stood for ejaculation. If a man
withheld his ejaculation, it was said that 'no rain
came', which meant that he could prolong lovemaking to indulge his beloved with the ultimate gift
of 'soaring clouds' – a rolling, lifting, flying orgasmic
high.

As the clouds soar, Huang O feels flowers of fire
blossoming inside her. Fireworks, with their
spectacular sequence of colourful explosions in the
heavens, were an invention of the ancient Chinese,
and the breathtaking displays that she witnessed at
court would have reminded the poet of the
exquisite orgasmic pleasure her lover gave her with
his tongue. The English word for this delicate art,
cunnilingus, sounds clinical and mundane compared to the many delightful traditional Chinese
terms, such as 'lotus-eating' or the more elaborate

'butterfly nibbling at the calyx of the flower', which express the act with poetic subtlety.

In addition to the ecstasy it gave to a woman, Chinese alchemists of sex believed that the delicious practice of lotus-eating was essential for the good health and well-being of her lover. A woman's body was the source of three precious yin fluids, potent elixirs for every man. The yang energies of the male rise like fire and radiate outwards to infinity; they are dynamic and forceful but need the nourishing, earthy yin energies of the female to ground and strengthen them. Likewise, the female needs the linear yang energy of the male to charge her and fire her up. Yin and yang capture and release each other like the two halves of a circle, refreshing and renewing the life force they generate between them.

To imbibe the restorative yin fluids of his beloved, a man was advised to drink from her Three Fountains. He sucked saliva from the Red Lotus Fountain of her lips when they kissed. He tasted milk, or its essence, a colourless fluid called

White Snow, from the Twin Lotus Fountains of her breasts as he nuzzled and suckled them. And in the most intimate and potent kiss of all, he drank the juices of love from the Purple Agaric Fountain as his tongue thrillingly explored the secret folds of her yoni to give her flowers of fire. The third fountain was so named because the clitoris was said to resemble the most highly valued of the five varieties of divine mushrooms, the purple-stalked agaric toadstool, not only in its appearance, but also in its power to give men a taste of eternity.

Drinking the heavenly essence from the beloved's Purple Agaric Fountain was considered to be a rare and heady experience worthy of great sacrifice. The sixth-century poet Hsu-Ling wrote to congratulate a friend who had given up his life at court and retired to live in the mountains with his concubine, enthusing, 'Why bother with the elixir of immortality when you can drink at the Jade Fountain!' (Yet another name for the yoni!) The art of the tongue was highly valued by the female sex for the power it gave them as well as the pleasure. The Empress Wu Hu, who reigned during the T'ang dynasty (CE 700–900), went so far as to issue a decree obliging all government officials and visiting dignitaries to pay homage to her royal person by drinking from her Jade Fountain. And such were the benefits of tasting the yin essence of an empress that courtiers and foreign visitors were willing to perform this intimate act in public. Scroll paintings depict the beautiful empress standing holding her robe open, while a high official kneels before her devotedly applying his lips and tongue to her yoni.

Certain fruits that are delicious to suck and eat have always suggested the delectable art of the tongue to the imagination of those who love to give or receive it. Wherever it is grown and enjoyed, the fig is a reminder of the intimate details of female sexual anatomy. Hidden inside the soft outer body, the ripe fruit is blood red, moist, honey–sweet and succulent. The dark glittering flesh strongly re–sembles the secret chamber of the yoni; the luscious taste of a fig warm in the hand from the sun, and the sight of its countless tiny seeds add to its potency as a symbol of female sexuality and fertility.

Across East Asia the fig with its sensual yoni–fruit is the tree that majestically links heaven and earth; from its roots to the tips of its branches it embodies the human life force rising from the earthy sensuality of the base chakra to the spiritual glory of the crown. The Buddha was sitting under a holy fig (*Ficus religiosa*), otherwise known as the Bodhi Tree or tree of Wisdom, when he attained enlightenment. But in the Judaeo–Christian tradition the sacred knowledge that the fig imparts was regarded with fear. The Genesis story tells how once Adam and Eve had understood their naked-ness, they were ashamed, and sewed fig leaves together to make aprons. Their choice of leaves only revealed what they were trying to conceal, suggest-ing that it was particularly the knowledge of female sexuality that was forbidden by the Old Testament God and his patriarchs.

For King Solomon – exceptional among biblical heroes in his celebration of sensuality – the pomegranate was an even more overtly sexual fruit than the fig. Pomegranate means apple of abundant grains or seeds, and its biblical name *rimon* comes from *rim*, 'to bear a child'. (In Latin, *rima* is the yonic cleft.) Solomon had pomegranates carved on the pillars of his temple as symbols of fertility. He also grew them to serve at his table. The beautiful rose-gold outer case of the pomegranate, like a giant rosehip, is cut open to reveal glistening rubies, the fruity coating of many seeds, nestling in a honey-comb of pithy membranes. The pomegranate is like a jewel box. Eating it is a delicate business, for once the ruby fruitlets have been removed from their casket, it requires skilful manoeuvring of tongue and lips to suck the sharply sweet and juicy fruit pulp from the seeds, which are usually spat out. The rare character of the fruit, its rich ruby colour and the subtle mouth movements required to enjoy it are all reminiscent of the intimate yonic kiss.

Solomon's bride invited him to drink the juice of her pomegranate and become her Lord of the Pomegranate, Baal–Rimon:

> *I would lead thee, and bring thee into my*
> *mother's house, who would instruct me: I*
> *would cause thee to drink of spiced wine of the*
> *juice of my pomegranate.*
>
> Song of Songs 8:2

The pomegranate, the fig, the purple agaric and the lotus blossom ... When these precious fruits of the earth are licked and sucked, toyed with by the tongue and nibbled at with the lips, they produce in man and woman an ecstasy so divine that it was thought by many ancient societies to bestow mystical powers of longevity, authority and creativity. By drinking the juices from the chalice of her yoni a woman's lover could gain the status of a god.

In Tantra, the religion of sex, the art of lotus–eating was called the Holy Kiss, because it was the gateway to both sexual ecstasy and spiritual enlightenment. This kiss was central to Maharutti, the Great Rite of Tantra. Initiates gathered in the temple of the goddess Kali, a womb–like cave lit by flares where her image was housed. Erotic incense hung heavily in the air. Sacrificial animals were led to the shrine, their throats cut and their blood collected in special vessels. Then the blood was poured through the yoni of the squatting goddess to anoint the phallus of her consort Shiva, as he lay beneath her. This act symbolized the union of male and female essences: the white semen, *sukra*, and the red menstrual blood, *rakta*. The priest and priestess representing Shiva and Kali tasted the sanctified blood, which was said to empower them and bring them to enlightenment. Then they re-enacted the rite in front of the worshippers, the priest on his back, the priestess squatting over his erect lingam and moving with abandon until he ejaculated inside her. At the climax of the rite the priestess parted her thighs and the priest lapped their mingled essences from her yoni, driving her wild with his lips and tongue. To complete the circle he kissed her mouth so that she too could taste the holy fluids. Excited and aroused by witnessing the Holy Kiss, the worshippers joined in the orgy. When all had performed the Great Rite, the sacrificed animals were cooked and eaten and washed down with quantities of wine.

The Tantrics performed the Holy Kiss whether a woman was menstruating or not. Indeed, to the ancients the love juices of the yoni were symbolic of the female essence that manifested in 'moon blood'. The mysterious blood that a woman shed according to the moon's phases was revered as divine. It was widely believed in ancient societies – and still taught in European medical schools up to the eighteenth century – that babies were created when moon blood remained in the womb and 'coagulated' into a new being. Men regarded this blood with holy awe and dread. The experience of this inexplicable miracle embodied in woman was forever denied them, except by tasting. Their ambivalent feelings about the exclusivity of its power led men to call this blood 'sacred', which in many languages has the original double meaning of both pure and impure, blessed and accursed – this blood was the primal taboo.

As well as carrying the potential for new life, moon blood was believed to transmit wisdom, both inherited from previous generations and divinely inspired. In many cultures a future king had to be initiated into the wisdom of the goddess by lapping moon blood at the yoni of her high priestess before he could be crowned. According to an ancient belief post-menopausal women are the wisest of all mortals, because they are no longer losing the blood that is the source of all wisdom. This is why they were called witches, meaning 'women of wit'. Their 'wise blood' was thought to give them super-natural powers; it made them feared by Christian society and was the cause of their persecution in medieval Europe.

As we have already discovered, in the early Middle Ages knowledge of Tantra filtered into Europe, carried by wandering minstrels called troubadours. They came originally from southern Spain, where they had learned from the Moorish conquerors of Andalucía Arabian love songs and poetry that celebrated the goddess incarnate in every woman. This Tantric principle – woman as goddess – became the cornerstone of a movement known as Courtly Love, or Romance. The troubadours travelled up through France and across northern Europe, entertaining knights and ladies at court after court with their stories. They sang of a beloved so noble and true that she was set apart from ordinary mortals; though unattainable, she could bestow on a man who proved himself worthy a love that would transform their lives with ecstatic illumination. The love of an unattainable woman ... ecstatic illumination ... it sounded like the cult of the Virgin Mary, which was enjoying a feverish popularity at the time, yet was its very antithesis. The revolution of Courtly Love was that the object of worship was a living flesh–and–blood woman and the way she was worshipped had nothing to do with the Church and its denial of earthly pleasures. Like Tantra itself, Courtly Love was a heady fusion of the spiritual and the sexual. Practised in private by an upper-class elite, it flowed like an underground river, running completely counter to mainstream Christian society with its male hierarchy and its virgin queen.

The beloved of medieval Romance was unattainable because she was already married. But from her pedestal of virtuous wedlock, she inspired a sexual passion that drove her lover to test himself to the limit in order to win her love. While the knight risked life and limb in jousting for her favour, the Lady also risked all – her status, her reputation, and even death – in keeping faith with him and agreeing to meet him in secret. Courtly Love was always adulterous, yet though it threatened to undermine marriage, it also depended on it. While marriage was the economic and political rock on which society was built, determining the inheritance of wealth and land and the allegiance of power, the passion of Courtly Love was fundamentally anti-social. Precisely because it had no status or recognition it was without duty and obligation and therefore burned pure and true to itself.

The restrictions of marriage only fuelled the lovers' desire. The obstacles in their path served to heighten the urgency of their resolve to reach each other. And when at last they did come together, there were still more restrictions to fire their passion. Because the essence of their love was freedom, lovers could not risk pregnancy, which might complicate loyalties or result in disgrace or death, so the code of courtly love forbade intercourse; yet there were more intimate ways in which they could enjoy each other. The clue lay in the name given to the archetypal fictional hero of medieval Romance, Tristan. Reverse the syllables to reveal his secret: *Tantris*. In the story of *Tristan and Isolde*, the heroine vows that no man has ever touched her between her legs except her husband Mark and the beggar who carried her across the river. Of course the reader knows that the beggar was none other than Tristan in disguise, and that she rode upon his shoulders. Isolde is speaking the truth, for the man's head was indeed between her legs.

The Holy Kiss was the consummation that courtly lovers dreamed of, the goal of their voyage of discovery. And the Holy Grail, the mythic chalice of the medieval romantic quest, was none other than the divine yoni of the beloved; it was said to overflow with the wine of enlightenment that inspired poets and sages. There was no greater love or homage a knight could pay to his Lady than to drink at her chalice, which was his ultimate reward.

The Holy Kiss is the sixth gateway to sexual bliss. To give the Holy Kiss signifies total acceptance; to receive it shows complete trust. For a woman, the tongue offers the perfect touch to release flowers of fire inside her: delicate, firm, precise, slippery, warm, generous, thrilling. And because it doesn't involve the penis, this caress feels like a gift. An act far more personal than penetration, its generosity liberates body and soul, like clouds soaring across the sky.

The man who gives the Holy Kiss can come to know his beloved in her most intimate nature, gaining a knowledge of her sexuality that is more secret, even, than her knowledge of herself. Sure of giving her exquisite pleasure that his hands and penis cannot match, he can relax into the kiss without a care for the reliability of his erection, immersing himself in her private world. He can take his time to enjoy the fascinating look of her genitals as they redden, unfold and swell. The feel of her skin on his face, the wetness of her on his lips as he buries his mouth in her yoni. The erotic scents and the sweet salty taste; the thick sexy feeling on his tongue. The rough and slippery textures that his tongue explores; the secret ridges, hollows and crevices. He can half dream with his lips on the softest parts of her, her thighs against his ears so he hears the blood thudding in her body. This depth of sensual knowledge is exhilarating, awe–inspiring, spiritual.

The
Conversation

'Her breath is like honey spiced
with cloves,
Her mouth delicious as a ripened
mango.
To press kisses on her skin is to
taste the lotus . . .'

THE CAVE ENGULFED THEM, ENDLESSLY DEEP and wide. In this world of infinite night there was no sound except echoing drips of water from above and the purling wash of their fragile craft as the ferryman pushed them onwards against the current with his long bamboo pole. Dwarfed by the awesome immensity of the cavern, Adam and the three courtesans sat spellbound and motionless in the tiny boat of split bamboo; at the prow, Padmini held aloft a torch of fire. In its undulating flame they saw huge stalactites glowing with luminous minerals, shining pinks and greens shot through with trickles of sulphur yellow, glittering ochre, deepest rust. The flame skittered across the mighty river that stretched its fingers into far-off underground tunnels; the wine-dark water rippled, sending spangles of indigo light to catch the iridescent colours in the rock. Grotesque shadows played gigantically across the miraculous stone icicles and the streaming walls of the cave, and a jagged dance of coloured reflections passed across the mesmerized faces of the travellers; only the hooded ferryman remained immune to the dazzling spectacle as he set his course upstream.

Eventually they drew up at a natural platform in the rock and the ferryman signalled to them to disembark. Adam helped his companions onto the narrow ledge. Picking her way gingerly around pools of agate and rose, Padmini led the party through a narrow passageway; stumbling, they followed the erratic flare of the torch into a marvellous grotto. There she held the torch up high and in its wavering light their eyes picked out a deep pool fed by a bubbling and steaming underground spring: the source of the great river. They saw a niche in the rock beyond the boiling spring, its walls pink and streaked with red, glistening and peaking into many folds, a royal canopy. On the bed below the canopy, a figure stirred. They moved closer through the whirling steam, hardly daring to breathe. A woman lay on her side with her left hand cupping her ear and her right hand cupping her genitals. She seemed to be dreaming. She wore a shift of scarlet shot through with purple and gold, diamonds blazed at her throat and in her hair.

As they stood and gazed at the sleeping figure, Padmini in a low voice recited a poem:

> *Her breath is like honey spiced with cloves,*
> *Her mouth delicious as a ripened mango.*
> *To press kisses on her skin is to taste the lotus,*
> *The deep cave of her navel hides a store of spices*
> *What pleasure lies beyond, the tongue knows,*
> *But cannot speak of it.*

Padmini turned to Adam, her eyes glowing in the torchlight. 'This is Lilith,' she whispered, 'the priestess of the great goddess Kali.' But Adam already knew. He had recognized her at once. Lila, his first wife, the diamond of the lotus flower, unchanged from the moment they had first met. Lilith opened her eyes and stared straight into his. 'Welcome, Adam,' she said. 'I have been expecting you.' She directed Padmini to spread a tiger skin at her feet where they could sit and talk by the bubbling spring.

'Our object in coming to this glistening yonic cave,' said Padmini, 'is to learn the secrets of the Holy Kiss. Lilith speaks for the great goddess whose spirit lives in all women. Listen carefully, then go home and share your knowledge with Eve.'

'The Holy Kiss is the sixth step to heaven on the ladder of sexual bliss,' said Lilith. 'Travellers on the path to the Seventh Heaven are forbidden inter-course, a restriction that is bound to inflame your desire for one another and suggest in your fantasies many more imaginative ways of satisfying it.

'The Holy Kiss offers the surest path to blissful orgasmic release for a woman; for a man, it is the most lavish expression of his adoration and lust. But it is more than that. One of the themes of the Seventh Heaven is respect for the individuality of your partner, and this depends on keeping a sense of separation between the two of you. In penetrative sex, lovers merge and become one; their individuality is lost. Over time, lovers who live together may even cease to see one another. The Seventh Heaven asks you to take a step back and refocus on your lover. It favours the Holy Kiss above all other caresses for a woman because the Kiss does not conquer or possess, but is an act of worship that sets the beloved free.'

'The mouth and the genitals are the two areas of the body most richly supplied with sensitive nerve endings,' explained Koriko. 'So when they come together during lovemaking the sensation is the most exquisite of all sexual pleasures. The art of the Holy Kiss is perfected through imaginative movements of the lips and tongue and intuitive understanding of your beloved's response.'

'Can you recommend any exercises for my lips and tongue?' asked Adam.

'My lover practised by eating ripe fresh figs,' said Padmini with a smile. 'He held the fig by the stalk and opened it from the top, splitting it into four. Then slowly and lasciviously he took off the rosy flesh with his lips. He did this for me to see.'

'In Japan gigolos used to exercise their lips and tongue by cracking and eating roasted melon seeds,' said Koriko. 'A champion of the art could toss a seed into his mouth, crack it with his teeth, separate the broken shell from the kernel with his tongue, spit out the shell and swallow the kernel, repeating the trick many times in lightning quick succession. Melon-seed cracking ensured a highly developed skill with mouth and tongue.'

'The best way to practise is on Eve herself,' said Marguerite. 'Practise the Kiss intensively as often as

Eve would like, and with minute attention to detail. This is how you will come to know your beloved intimately, her taste, her feel, her scent, which the French call *cassolette*, and her intimate responses. Thus you will learn how to perfect the art of setting her free on the soaring clouds of a rolling orgasmic high.'

Adam wondered whether Eve would get as much pleasure from the Kiss when she was menstruating as during the other three weeks of the month. He wondered too whether he would enjoy it then; he had never tasted her blood before.

'If she could relax into it, it would undoubtedly be a powerful experience for Eve,' said Lilith. 'Many women feel a special hunger for sex during their periods, particularly towards the end of the menstrual flow. At this time orgasm can provide a kind of sexual healing because it often relieves the cramp and backache that tend to accompany a period. A dark red towel placed under her hips can spare the sheets.'

'Many men enjoy it too,' said Marguerite. 'In fact in France, moon blood was thought to have aphrodisiac powers. Madame de Montespan vouched for its success with her lover Louis XIV. And it was the custom for a *lune de miel* or honeymoon to last a whole month – or moon – so that the bridegroom would have the chance to taste his bride's *honey*. That is how the honeymoon got its name.'

'Whether you taste the honey or not is unimportant,' said Koriko with a wave of her hand. 'But there is a lesson to be learned from this ancient custom – to honour moon blood for its part in the cyclical life force of humankind. In modern times men and women live too remotely from the natural world. They regard the monthly bleeding as an unpleasant inconvenience, and this cannot but reflect badly on a woman.'

'And now let us talk about relaxation, which is the key to Eve's pleasure,' said Lilith. 'The way to relaxation is to give your beloved unlimited amounts of time and attention. Only by losing track of time will you taste eternity.'

'So make sure she is comfortable,' said Marguerite, 'lying back among pillows or cushions, or sitting in a deep armchair with her legs open, and resting on the arms...'

'There are many positions to try,' said Lilith, 'and no reason why you shouldn't experiment with more than one of them in a single session. It can add urgency and excitement to change position. Whatever position you choose, the sensation in her Coral Grotto will be heavenly.'

'You could start with Eve kneeling on all fours facing away from you,' said Koriko, edging away from the bubbling spring, which seemed to be getting hotter. 'The only disadvantage for her is that there's no one to kiss, hold and hug, so keep your hands on her body all the time, stroke her belly, perhaps even hold her hand.'

'How about lying side by side in the sixty-nine position?' Adam wanted to know.

Lilith shook her head. 'It is impossible to concentrate on two sensations at once. You may think you can, but what happens is that your attention flicks rapidly between the two. It is distracting. It is far better to immerse yourself fully in each sensation, first giving, then receiving. Only then will you be able to relax into the luxury of intimate timing and response.'

Koriko agreed. 'By all means lie head to toe on your sides. But put no pressure on Eve to pay attention to your Jade Stalk. Suggest that she merely cradles it in her hand while you lick her. She can gaze at it and dream, sometimes gently fondling it or touching it with the tip of her tongue, but for the most powerful orgasm she should do nothing to detract from the sensations you are giving her. Besides, it can be dangerous for you if your tender part is between her teeth when she comes . . .'

'There is another way of eating the lotus,' said Lilith. 'It was beloved of Kali, who always took the more active role when making love to Shiva. She liked him to lie down so that she could squat with her yoni over his mouth. Many women fantasize about this position, but are reluctant to suggest it for fear of seeming too dominant. So ask Eve if she would like to try it.

'She can steady herself by holding onto the head of the bed while you rest your head on a pillow and offer her your open mouth and tongue. She then takes charge, dipping down to receive your touch and moving against you. It is strenuous for your tongue, so you may want to change positions after a while, but it is a very good education in which parts of her yoni she likes to be stimulated, as well as in the pace and pressure she most enjoys. You can help by cupping her buttocks in your hands, or reach up to fondle her breasts.'

'Or of course you could try the Kiss by kneeling in front of Eve as she stands there holding her robe open like the Chinese Empress Wu Hu,' said Koriko. 'You could pretend to be her servant.' She threw Adam a wicked smile.

'If you had ever experienced the delight of lotus-eating on a swing you would shiver with ecstasy at the memory of it,' exclaimed Padmini. 'Oh, the delight of being nudged through the air by your lover's tongue, and of being able to keep just the right balance and pressure by leaning in to him, or pushing away from him with the slightest movement of your toes on his shoulders!'

'That sounds like heaven indeed,' sighed Lilith, her eyes shining. 'A Kiss that really does make a woman fly!'

'And deliciously tantalizing for the man,' said Padmini. 'My lover said my yoni was as fragrant and beautiful as a peony flower and it reminded him of dipping his head among its delicate mass of pink petals.'

'Every woman has her own unique *cassolette*, her intimate scent,' said Marguerite. 'After you have tasted her, appreciate her juices on your fingers and lips. There is nothing more flattering for a woman than to know her lover finds her delicious.'

'But we are running ahead of ourselves!' said Lilith. 'Make sure you thoroughly awaken Eve's desires before touching her yoni with your tongue. Remember the yoni rub, and how to cup her whole yoni in your palm and give it the firm and reassuring warmth of your hand while it is still closed, which will make it long to be touched inside. Breathe hot air onto the delicate skin of her inner thighs, kiss and caress them to tantalize her desires.'

'Then kiss and nuzzle at the yoni,' said Koriko. 'Peel back the outer lips with your lips and fingers – as if it were a ripe fig – and hold Eve's secret parts open, or let her do this for you. Or the Coral Grotto may already be pushed open by its own excitement.'

The cave grew steamier. 'Explore the outer lips of her yoni–fruit first,' said Lilith silkily, as her diamonds flashed at her throat. 'Outline the shape, find the grooves with your tongue and run the tip lightly along them, up and back again. Flicking and licking. Lasciviously press the flat of your tongue against the moist red hills. Run the tip along the central valley, tickling the Golden Gulley above, the Jade Vein below, and the round hole of the Jade Gate in between the two.'

'Keep your touch light and well lubricated,' said Padmini. 'Eve will let you know when she wants firmer pressure by straining her yoni towards you. Saliva is the best lubricant of all, but if you have been playing with her using almond oil, you won't find the taste unpleasant.'

'Let the excitement build before you touch her Diamond,' said Koriko, breathing heavily in the humid air. 'Let your tongue play for a while in the Divine Field, the exquisitely sensitive area above the Diamond, so that you approach it from the hooded side. Circle the Diamond with the tip of your tongue. If she is very sensitive, she may only want you to touch it through the hood, or at the root or perhaps at the Lute Strings. With your face so close, you will be able to marvel at all the mysterious details of her anatomy and come to know her response as intimately as if it were your own. The Diamond may disappear inside its hood to protect it against too much stimulation, but this does not mean you should stop tonguing the yoni.'

Marguerite said, 'Touch her Diamond occasionally – move your head quickly left to right across it a number of times. The art is to keep excitement at a high plateau and not to rush or over-stimulate, which will break the blissful trance she is in. Keep control by tantalizing her – this way her excitement will mount of its own accord and she will always be wanting more. She is your goddess – let her lead the way.'

'Give her time and more time,' said Lilith. 'Only when she is thoroughly relaxed in the confidence that you are not going to stop until she comes, however long that takes, will she allow herself to become completely absorbed in sensation and carried away on the rhythm of your licking. To stop your tongue getting tired, use your nose and your chin as well as your mouth, so as you move up and down, you stimulate her with all three points. (Make sure you have shaved smoothly before you make love as stubble can tear the tender flesh of the yoni.) And make the most of the long strokes by moving your head and keeping your tongue still, letting it rest by your bottom lip rather than sticking it out, which certainly can be very tiring. For left-to-right strokes, stick your tongue out and keep it still while you move your head, saving your tongue muscles for the rapid flicking strokes that women love so much.'

'My lover used to write love messages across my yoni with his tongue', confided Marguerite. 'And I would find it very erotic to hear the lapping and licking sounds his tongue made. Mouth music was our name for it.'

'Your tongue is a much more potent weapon in the armoury of love than your Jade Stalk, you know, Adam', said Koriko. 'It offers the surest way of bringing Eve to bliss and it is always reliable and responsive to your every command. As you proceed, take note of every stage in her arousal, so you can move with the build-up to her climax. You already know what to look for. The swollen and reddened fruit of her yoni will be glistening with love juice mingled with your own saliva – the more saliva you make, the more excitingly slippery your tongue will feel. Keep contact with her body with your hands, gently stroke and tease her inner thighs, sweep your palm across her belly, touch her breasts, squeeze her hand, feel the huge pulse of love at the arteries in her groin. Imagine you are a butterfly or a bee, hovering at her Jade Gate suspended by your wings, sipping at the bud of the night-blooming jasmine, opening it with the tip of your tongue greedy for its juice. The most delicate movements will send her spiralling into orgasm. See how long you can make her last without tipping over the edge.'

'As the climax nears and she begins to strain and gasp, she may want you to apply firmness. You can use your fingers as well,' said Lilith, fanning herself with a peacock feather fan. 'It can be very sexy to give her your finger to suck. Some like a finger just inside the Jade Gate. A powerful point to press is the Stairway to Heaven, the midpoint on the perineum. Or put one of *her* fingers in your mouth, so that it gets mixed up with what you are doing with your tongue. If she finds fingers a distraction, cup both her buttocks firmly in your hands as you thrust your tongue inside the Jade Gate and flick its rim.'

'As her body tenses, keep up a rapid and firm flicking movement with your tongue,' said Padmini. 'At the first convulsion, press the flat of your tongue *hard* along the valley of the yoni and keep it there until she has subsided.'

'Or suck vigorously on the Diamond!' cried Lilith with shining eyes.

'Or thrust your tongue as far as you can into her Jade Gate,' sighed Koriko.

'Or drag your tongue firmly up and down the whole length of the overripe yoni as you hold her legs firmly apart and she clamps them round your ears', breathed Marguerite.

They sat for a few moments in a silence punctuated only by the bubbling of the spring. 'The moments after orgasm are so precious for a woman,' said Padmini. 'She needs to be held and loved so that she can truly feel the emotions you have released in her.'

'Kiss her on the mouth,' said Lilith, 'and let her revel in her own scents and juices. Ask her if she wants more ...'

In the torchlight, through the gradually dispersing steam, the colours of the grotto were clear and beautiful once more.

SCROLL 7

The Jade Pillar

❧

The Courtesans' Parchment

The ancients were far ahead of the modern world in their understanding of sexuality, and their wisdom still has plenty to teach us.

*I*N ANCIENT TIMES THE PHALLUS WAS worshipped for its miraculous power to rise from the dead. Its death and resurrection mirrored the other great cyclical mysteries of nature – the sunrise and sunset, the revolving seasons and the harvest – and seemed to offer striking proof that divinity and immortality were embodied in every man. The world's oldest mythologies were built on the mystique of male sexual potency. The first stories ever written celebrate a heroic god who suffers, dies and rises again, bringing his people salvation and eternal life through the power of his penis.

The Egyptians told the story of Osiris and Isis, the

incestuous brother and sister who were king and queen in the first age of the world. Osiris was a gentle teacher who civilized his people and showed them how to grow crops on the rich flood plains of the Nile; Isis invented weaving and healed the sick with medicinal plants. But their brother Set was jealous of their success. In the twenty-eighth year of Osiris's life he secretly measured the king's body and had a marvellous sarcophagus made to his exact dimensions. Then he held a feast at which he offered the beautifully decorated tomb to anyone whom it would fit. One by the one the guests climbed in to try it for size. Finally, suspecting nothing, Osiris lay down inside it; instantly Set's men nailed on the lid and poured boiling lead over it to seal it tight. Then Set had the coffin cast adrift on the Nile. The waters of the great river dwindled, the crops died and the people starved.

When Isis heard of this treachery, she was stricken with grief. She knew that the dead cannot rest until their bodies have been buried with proper funeral rites, so she set out to find her husband's corpse. She found the sarcophagus in a faraway land, lodged by the river in a tamarind tree. Isis brought the coffin home and opened it to begin her mourning, but when Set discovered the body, he hacked it into fourteen pieces and strewed them about the kingdom. The sacred lunar number fourteen signified the number of steps on Osiris's mystic ladder. For fourteen days the dead king descended into the Underworld; it took him another fourteen days to rise again. Meanwhile, his distraught queen searched Egypt for his remains and managed to recover all of them except his penis. On the twenty-eighth day she bound Osiris into a whole, creating the first mummy. Then she made a new phallus out of clay or, in another version of the story, turned herself into a hawk and hovered over the groin of the dead king until by her power a new phallus arose. Isis lowered herself onto it; as Osiris ejaculated, the Nile flooded and made the land fertile once more.

The story of the phallic god and his promise of eternal life runs deep in the mythic imagination. The Greek saviour and god of the harvest, Adonis, was gored in the groin by the goddess of love disguised as a bull, then his severed phallus was buried in a cave, where it grew into his son, Priapus. Priapus was a small god, dwarfed by the immensity of his perpetual erection. The Roman saviour Attis was also castrated, then crucified on a pine tree; his holy blood poured down to fertilize and redeem the earth. All these stories fed into the story of Jesus, which shares the same essential phallic elements of suffering, death and rebirth.

For worshippers of the phallus, its shape took on magic powers. Standing stones in the landscape, carved obelisks, sceptres carried as symbols of authority by priests or kings, all were imbued with sexual potency. In India pillars were erected in honour of Shiva's sacred lingam; they became popular pilgrimage sites. The land around the pillar was known as the Kingdom of Shiva, a place of miracles, and anyone who stepped into it would receive instant remission of sins. Like all Eastern gods, Shiva was called 'Christ', which means 'anointed' and comes from the practice of anointing the divine phallus – sometimes euphemistically called his 'head' – with holy oil, wine or blood in preparation for the sacred marriage bed. If a woman wished to conceive, she rubbed the head of Shiva's reddened lingam with her finger and whispered a prayer. Shiva's festivals were celebrated with a fertility dance around a maypole hung with streaming red and white ribbons. Men danced clockwise around the phallic pole and women anti-clockwise, weaving in and out. The women held the red ribbons to symbolize their menstrual blood; the men held the white ribbons, the colour of semen. As they danced, the ribbons plaited together at the top of the pole, uniting to create new life.

In the Greek empire riotous springtime cel-ebrations marked the rising of the sap with the raising of a monumental phallus. At a festival in

Alexandria in 270 BCE a golden phallus of astonishing length (one hundred and eighty feet), with a gold star at the tip, was paraded through ecstatic crowds as poems were sung in praise of Dionysus, another saviour god. Heading the procession were ten rows of ostriches ridden by boys dressed as satyrs, scores of Ethiopians bearing elephant tusks, dozens of peacocks, sixteen cheetahs, fourteen leopards, a white bear, a rhino and a giraffe. A gilded statue of Zeus, the divine father of Dionysus, and fifty thousand foot soldiers followed behind.

The proudly erect phallus was used in the ancient world to stake out territories and warn off intruders. The Greeks marked their boundaries with phalluses of stone or wood called herms, which they also erected in conquered lands to show possession. Named after Hermes, god of fertility and prosperity, they featured his head on top of a plain pillar with a realistic erect penis carved at the front. Hermes guaranteed the success of all sorts of undertakings. One of his jobs was to guide travellers, so herms sprang up at crossroads as well as at public and private doorways, where they exercised a protective function and brought good luck.

The luck of ancient Rome was invested in Priapus. Statues of the diminutive god with the oversized phallus were installed around properties to advertise ownership and keep out trespassers. Adolescent boys were given a *bulla*, a locket to be worn around the neck, inside which was a lucky charm – a priapic phallus called a *fascinum*. The development of this word to its modern meaning shows the awesome and intriguing power that the male organ can exert on the mind. Looking at the little charm may have inspired the wet dreams of puberty that were such a cause of rejoicing in ancient Rome, where citizens celebrated their sons' first ejaculation at a state holiday called Liberalia.

The spirit of the phallus was publicly worshipped and fêted, but like any other god, it needed to be nurtured and placated, because in private it did not always fulfil man's fantasies and dreams. There is probably no man in history who has not worried at least fleetingly about size. And as long as there has been insecurity about the size of the penis, there have been ingenious ways of making it look and feel bigger.

The practice of dressing the penis stretches back into prehistory. In a six-thousand-year-old grave at Varna on the Bulgarian Black Sea coast, a skeleton was found adorned with many beautiful metal objects. Between its legs was a fine gold sheath, shaped to fit snugly onto an erect penis, with a hole at the tip and perforations around the rim. It could have been sewn onto a garment made of cloth or leather, or even onto the skin of the penis itself. It might have been used in a fertility rite, or padded like a codpiece for ceremonial wear. But the most interesting speculation is that it was placed on the body after death, giving a man of stature a golden penis that would make him immortal by rising again in the afterworld.

Where nakedness is vulnerability, clothing is power. A limp penis is not as intriguing as a golden sheath, or even a fig leaf – or the Dionysian vine leaf seen in most works of art – which draws attention and imaginative speculation to what it conceals. The male *cache-sexe* can be as obvious as a loincloth or a codpiece or as obscure as a sporran, the traditional Scots purse decorated with hairy tassels that hangs outside the kilt. Eye–catching penis sheaths are commonly worn in the tribal communities of the tropics by men who wear very little else. The warrior's costume of Irian Jaya features a stout bamboo phallus that reaches almost to the chin. It is secured with ties under the buttocks and again at the middle around the waist. The purpose of all these dressings is to symbolize masculinity while keeping the real state of the penis private.

Kokigami, the Japanese 'art of the little paper costume', is probably the most sophisticated form of penis dressing ever invented. Directness is un-welcome to the Japanese, whose sensitivities lead them rather towards symbolism, mystery and restraint. Hence when gifts are given, it is considered impolite to hand them over unwrapped, and packaging was long ago turned into a fine art called *tsutsumi*. The word means 'discretion' or 'modesty'.

In a nation skilled at wrapping gifts, it was only natural that a man should wrap his erect penis before presenting the gift of love. The *Kojiki*, a book of legends dating from CE 712, contains several stories that relate how men would wrap their penises in silks and ribbons or even seaweed before retiring to the conjugal chamber. The more complicated the wrappings and the longer the wife took to unwrap them with her delicate fingers, the more delicious the mounting excitement for both. This elegant intimate practice was the forerunner of *kokigami*. When Buddhism arrived in Japan in the sixth century, Shinto priests sought ways of

controlling sexual energy with the mind, transcend-
ing the purely physical aspects of sex and
heightening satisfaction. Instead of simply binding
then releasing the penis, little paper costumes were
beautifully painted and cut for it in the shapes of
animals such as dragons, tigers and pigs, each
suggesting its own personality that could be
developed by the wearer and his partner into a
play. Through these costumes the ancient Shinto
beliefs in the divinity of the phallus took on a new
dimension.

During the Heian period (794–1185), Japan's
golden age of artistic development, *kokigami* was
adopted as a path to sensual enlightenment among
the upper classes. Erotic prints show couples
absorbed in enacting the drama of the *koki*.
Still popular today, it is an ingenious game for
lovers who wish to experiment with their sexual
fantasies.

Most mammals, including many primates, are equipped with a penile bone called a baculum or *os penis*. But not man. Coaxing the reluctant penis was one of the first aims of developing medicine in the ancient world, where the unreliability of the human erection led to the early invention of aphrodisiacs. While some specially prescribed foods and herbs were subtly effective when taken regularly over a long period of time, other treatments relied on superstition or the gullibility of the client. Into this last category fell a variety of magic remedies made from animal parts, such as badger testicles, ant juice, rendered–down camel humps, the penises of swans, tigers and asses, the teeth and tails of crocodiles, deer antlers, frogs' bones, goats' eyes, snails' necks, and a broth made of vipers. The search for the invincible phallic horn gave rise to the myth of the unicorn, a magnificent white horse with a single horn growing from the top of its head. The unicorn was said to be impossible to capture, but if a virgin sat down in the forest to rest, the proud creature would lie next to her and fall into an enchanted sleep with its head in her lap. Huntsmen could then creep out of the undergrowth and saw off the horn without harming the beast.

Perhaps the most famous and least understood of animal aphrodisiacs is Spanish fly, the common name of the beetle *Lytta vesicatoria*. Clay tablets from ancient Iraq reveal that Spanish fly was being recommended by Assyrian physicians three thousand years ago. The beetles are dried and crushed to extract the active ingredient, cantharis. When swallowed, this causes an intense burning sensation in the mouth and throat, followed by diarrhoea and the passing of blood in the urine. Then the urogenital tract becomes inflamed and bursts into blisters, making urination impossible. A side-effect is an engorged and throbbing penis, due not so much to sexual urgency as to excruciating pain. Dangerously toxic minerals such as mercury and arsenic were also used as irritants to produce instant erections.

Food and sex are natural companions in hunger, sensual pleasure and satisfaction, and in the blurring of kissing, biting and eating; a feast is the traditional prelude to love. Highly nutritious foods, such as honey, eggs and milk, were rightly prized for boosting sexual energy. The ancients knew that the libido depended on a healthy diet, something that lovers today – in an era of fast meals and processed foods – sometimes forget. In India a supper of poached sparrows' eggs was served on a bed of rice cooked in milk and drizzled with honey and melted butter. In Europe lovers stirred their honey into wine; in Arabia they spooned it onto crushed almonds and pine nuts. The Greeks ate shellfish to raise their libido, while the Vikings chewed garlic. Garlic was known to be good for the heart and believed to increase the supply of blood to the penis, as was ginger, which is also taken to improve the circulation. The Greeks wrapped slices of ginger root in a piece of bread and ate it to heat their blood before a night of love – the origin of the custom of giving gingerbread hearts as Valentines.

Every day the Aztec Emperor Montezuma drank fifty cups of hot chocolate to sustain his efforts in the harem, while Casanova diligently swallowed four dozen oysters. Chocolate is rich in phenyl-ethylalamine (PEA), a natural aphrodisiac produced in the brain by falling in love. Oysters, eaten raw, are full of active enzymes and hormones, and contain large amounts of zinc, which is vital for the healthy functioning of the prostate. In Bulgaria, Turkey and Japan, raw pumpkin seeds were eaten as a daily snack to preserve sexual potency; a hand-ful a day will do more than anything to protect a man's prostate gland from cancer and maintain its healthy functioning into advanced old age. All culinary herbs, spices and seasonings were known to be effective stimulants and excitants, as anyone who uses them regularly would soon discover on giving them up.

Many foods were sworn by for their power to induce lust. Some have always been relished for their suggestively sexual appearance and the unusually sensual experience of eating them: velvety-capped mushrooms that spring up overnight; downy-skinned peaches that run with nectar at the first bite. Eating the artichoke is a delicate matter – it can't be rushed at with a knife and fork and wolfed down in one or two mouthfuls. Instead, the delight of savouring this tantalizing vegetable is increased by admiration of its form, and by anticipation, as each leaf is pulled away individually and dipped in a rich buttery sauce. The plump, fleshy part of the leaf is eaten by a combination of nibbling and sucking. It requires total, relaxed concentration. When each leaf has been dealt with, the bristly choke has to be removed before the sublimely tender, delicately flavoured heart can be spooned onto the tongue. Eating asparagus spears involves fingers and lips, melted butter and eye contact, with lingering flirtatious excitement. Once the imagination is involved, all food has aphrodisiac potential. The Romans were even inspired by lettuces – they carried them in spring fertility parades because when they are cut they ooze a milky sap that looks not unlike semen.

Long ago in a remote and mountainous part of China, there lived a very observant goatherd. One day after he had moved his herd to new pasture, he noticed that the billy goats were frisking about and mounting and rutting with unusual enthusiasm. The goatherd soon realized that the animals' new-found energy came from nibbling excitedly at a certain patch of herbs. So he picked some of them and took them home. From then on, the goatherd drank a daily infusion of the weeds, and soon he could make love to his wife all night long. So he harvested his secret patch of herbs and went down the mountain to make his fortune, naming the plant *yin-yang-huo* – horny goat weed.

This ancient herb, which has the botanical name *Aceranthus sagittatum*, is one of the most potent male aphrodisiacs on earth. Around five thousand years ago the Chinese Emperor Shen Nung published a *Pharmacopoeia* in which he rated horny goat weed as highly as the best ginseng. Though the Chinese knew more powerful mineral aphrodisiacs, such as cinnabar and arsenic, they rightly believed that the habit of using strong drugs for instant effect the moment before they were needed would eventually lead to a burn-out of sexual potency. Instead the Emperor recommended that herbal tonics be carefully prescribed, measured and blended to suit each individual diagnosis and taken regularly, in small amounts, over a long period, a practice that continues today in traditional Chinese medicine. That way the aphrodisiac could be personalized, offering the right combination of stimulation with nourishment of the seminal or prostatic fluid, or the blood.

Because aphrodisiacs, when taken correctly, strengthen sexual tissues as well as increasing secretions of sex hormones, they enhance a man's control of his sexual response. They also increase the amount of semen lost at each ejaculation, making the preservation of semen even more important to Taoist lovers. The Taoists believed that while an active sex life was vital for health and longevity, semen should be retained by ejaculation control so that it could 'nourish the brain'. These ideas are not as absurd as they sound. Semen and the fluids of the brain and spinal cord consist of the same basic ingredients, so when semen is not ejaculated but reabsorbed into the soft tissues of the prostate, it will indeed indirectly 'nourish the brain'. And apart from the obvious benefits to health of love and happiness, sexual activity stimulates the production of hormones, which increase immunity to disease, offering the prospect of better health and a longer life, especially if the precious semen is not wasted.

The Taoist approach to sexual potency was holistic. Herbal tonics were just part of a balanced regime consisting of a nutritious diet, acupuncture, massage, and daily exercise to strengthen both stamina and breathing. Above all, they advocated moderation in everything. But just in case, the Chinese also invented a complete armoury of sex accessories – passion clips, passion ribbons and lust rings – to keep the Jade Pillar erect. The most common boudoir aid was the dragon ring, a ring of ivory designed to be worn around the base of the penis. A ribbon ran through a hole in the ring, under the scrotum and round the waist, where it was tied to keep it in place during loveplay. When the man contracted his pelvic floor muscles, causing the penis to swell, the ring exerted pressure on the veins, preventing loss of erection. It also pressed on the urogenital tract, helping him control his ejaculation.

The Taoists were never prudish about sex, simply regarding it as a natural, essential and healthy part of life, so over the centuries they studied the human sexual response with thoroughness and curiosity and recorded what they learned with reverence and accuracy. This approach was inconceivable in the moralistic West until about fifty years ago, and even then the scientists of sex presented their findings in a way that spoke of the laboratory rather than the bedroom. Thus the ancients were far ahead of the modern world in their understanding of sexuality, and their wisdom still has plenty to teach us.

The Conversation

Erotic skills have to be discovered, practised, cultivated and developed. They require attention and imagination.

*A*S THE COLOURFUL PROCESSION OF sedan chairs bearing the three courtesans and their students wound up the mountainside, a long skein of white cranes glided miraculously across the huge orange disc of the rising sun. Adam gazed after the magnificent birds as they followed the contours of the towering snow-capped peak on the other side of the valley.

At a signal from their leader the men set the sedan chairs gently on the ground. Koriko was in charge of this expedition. She had discarded her kimono in favour of a tunic and trousers lined against the chilly mountain air with the fur of the snow rabbit. Calling to the others to follow, she led them through the scrub to some steep steps hewn into the rock many centuries before, and well worn by pilgrims and travellers. As Eve climbed up after her, she noticed that the soles of Koriko's little felt shoes were embroidered with clouds.

Soon they came to a plateau dominated by a massive Pillar of Jade. Carved with ebullient realism, it loomed up in front of them, a touchingly enthusiastic monument to the yang power of masculinity, complete in every thrilling detail with rearing head and swollen veins that seemed to throb before their eyes.

'In the Orient,' said Koriko, smiling at her students' surprised expressions, 'the Jade Pillar has been an object of fascinated study for at least five thousand years, whereas most of your Western scientific knowledge of how it works has been gathered only over the past two centuries.'

Marguerite spread some rugs on the ground and invited them all to sit and contemplate the sculpture. 'It was once thought in the West that erections were governed by spirits (according to the Church, of course, they were caused by the Devil)', she explained, 'and that the penis swelled because it was filled with air. The Greeks called erection "inflation by wind". They believed a breath–like spirit arose in the liver, then moved on to the heart, before blowing through the arteries to fill the hollow organ of the penis. But of course the penis erects because sexual excitement sends blood rush–ing to fill the spongy tissues inside it.'

'In India we call the penis by its ancient Sanskrit name, the *lingam*,' said Padmini. 'It means "wand of light". I want you to look up at this magnificent Jade Pillar we see before us, and imagine that you hold it in your hand, a wand of light, a body of pure energy. So many lovers handle the lingam as though it were an inanimate tool, but if you are aware how alive it is as you stroke it and play with it, then it will live for you.'

'Knowing the intimate geography of the penis

will allow you to communicate very specific desires,' said Marguerite to Adam, 'and then Eve's love-making will become more detailed and attentive. So let us study it more closely. In your imagination, examine first the testicles. In most men, the left one is larger and hangs slightly lower than the right. A muscle called the dartos relaxes in hot weather to lower the testicles, and contracts in the cold to draw them closer to the body's warmth. Feel the testes gently in your fingers. Inside each one is an intricate bundle of fine tubes of astonishing length – seven hundred and fifty metres – that's nearly a mile of tubing for both testes! And in these tubes the sperm are produced. Sperm would not survive the body's heat, which is why the testicles hang outside it in the scrotum.'

'Of course our Oriental names are so much more poetic than the clinical terms Marguerite is using,' said Koriko. 'We call the testicles the Jade Balls; they nestle inside the Jade Pouch. The towering shaft of the penis with its swollen, rope-like veins, is the

Tree of Life; the vellum-smooth glans is the Velvet Head, or sometimes we call it the Turtle's Head. The opening at its tip, which you call the meatus, we have given the noble name of the Jade Gate. The fleshy lip of the corona is the Garland of Happiness; it runs like a collar beneath the Head and is gathered at the exquisitely sensitive frenulum, the narrow band of crinkled skin that we call the Lute Strings.

'In the Orient we have always known that erotic excitement begins in the mind, which is why we use such imaginative and playful language in the bedroom. It helps a man reach the Three Conditions for love. The first condition is desire. A man cannot make love against his will – and it furthers nothing to persuade him against his will. The second condition is relaxation. Only if a man is relaxed and confident will he be able to immerse himself fully in the depth and detail of lovemaking. The third condition is generosity. Only a generous lover will be able to truly satisfy his beloved and receive fulfilment in return. And when a man fulfils the Three Conditions for love, the Jade Stalk rises, and the Jade Balls are drawn up firmly at its root.'

'When you stroke the shaft of the penis,' said Marguerite, 'you will notice that the skin is extremely fine and elastic, thinner and looser than elsewhere in the body. Hold the shaft firmly in a relaxed fist and slowly and lightly move your fist up and down, so the skin glides smoothly over the shaft. Smooth, rhythmic stroking, and you feel the penis swelling, gradually getting harder and hotter in your hand. Invite the erection with a little pressure from your fingers and generous warmth from your palm; coax it, admire it, let it lead the way; never demand. See how the super-sensitive glans, the corona and the frenulum enlarge and swell, making them even more receptive to erotic sensation. Feel how the tissues inside the penis engorge with blood, squeezing shut the veins at the base and trapping the blood inside. Take pleasure in the thought that though the penis has fewer nerve endings than your hands or lips, the erotic stimulation you are giving it has the extraordinary power of being able to take over the brain.'

'It does completely take over the brain – and all the senses,' agreed Adam. 'But since that is so, why do I instantly lose my erection and all my sexual feelings if I hear a sudden noise – say the telephone rings?'

'The sudden interruption triggers the age-old instinct for self-preservation,' said Marguerite. 'Our male ancestors needed to react quickly if they were threatened or attacked in their most private moments. Evolution's survival tactic was to trigger the release of adrenaline, a hormone that immediately constricts the spongy tissue in the penis, releasing the veins and allowing the blood to flow quickly back into the body, so that the erection subsides. To avoid this happening, we recommend complete privacy and seclusion for lovemaking, and always advise unplugging the phone!

'When nothing happens to interrupt the erotic

swoon of the brain', she went on, 'the penis continues to respond to stimulation. Excitement mounts, and eventually the sperm move from the testes, along the vas deferens – the tube that is cauterized during a vasectomy to stop sperm mixing with the ejaculate – and up to the seminal glands and the prostate. These glands produce the fluid that makes up semen; they lie inside the body at the root of the penis. The prostate is the centre of orgasmic sensation. At the climax of excitement, the seminal glands and the prostate powerfully contract, squeezing shut the duct to the bladder as they pump out their precious fluids. These secretions mix with the sperm, and the semen is forced out of the penis by strong rhythmic contractions of the whole pelvic floor. Five hundred million sperm are ejaculated in less than a teaspoon of semen, and the orgasm lasts from two to ten seconds.'

'Western scientists with their fondness for statistics have analysed semen', said Koriko, 'and discovered that it contains thirty-two nutrients, including proteins, glucose, vitamins C and B12, sulphur, zinc and potassium. The ancients would not have been at all surprised by these findings. The Tantrics and Taoists taught men how to avoid ejaculating not just so they could prolong love-making, but to conserve semen and benefit from its highly nutritious qualities. The secrets of ejaculation control will soon be imparted to you.' She bowed to Adam, but his mind was busy with another worry.

'Talking of statistics,' he said, 'I have to ask whether the ancients placed any value on size – the size of the penis, that is.'

Koriko smiled. 'All men want to know the answer to this question; the Yellow Emperor himself asked it of his concubines. The truth is that while there will always be women who admire a Jade Stalk of tremendous proportions, common sense will tell you that size does not make a man a good lover. The true pleasure of sex has nothing whatever to do with external qualities. Erotic skills have to be discovered, practised, cultivated and developed. They require attention and imagination. You, Adam, are already highly skilled because you have progressed to the seventh gateway of the Seventh Heaven, the secret knowledge of the Jade Pillar, the subject of our present discussion.'

Eve said, 'You haven't mentioned the foreskin. Is there much difference between handling a circumcised penis and an uncircumcised one?'

'The foreskin is the loose hood of double skin that covers and protects the glans while the penis is at rest', said Marguerite. 'But it is also a continuation of the sheath of skin that covers the shaft of the penis. The special character of this skin is that it is fixed only at the root of the penis and below the coronal ridge. In between these points it is free to be stroked up and down the shaft and rolled in on itself over the glans in a sliding movement that creates intense pleasure. Circumcision is a cut at the coronal ridge that removes not just the hood–end of the foreskin, but also the excess of loose skin that glides so sensuously along the shaft.'

'So is a circumcised penis less sensitive?' asked Eve with a degree of concern.

'Scientific tests have proved there is no difference in sensitivity,' said Marguerite. 'The difference lies in the appearance and the manner of handling. Some women say a circumcised penis looks neater, while others love the sense of discovery that goes with rolling back the head of the foreskin to reveal the glans. Some find the uncircumcised penis easier to handle because of the way the loose skin glides on the shaft. With a circumcised member the skin on the shaft feels tauter and less mobile, so you may need to create more friction against your hand as you play with it. If you are ever uncertain, ask your lover to show you how he does it himself.'

'A woman can learn a lot by watching her lover,' said Padmini. 'Then she can improve on his repertoire by adding imaginative variations of her own.'

'And now let us turn to the whole delicious business of arousal,' said Koriko. 'We start with the extremities and move gradually inwards. In my training as a geisha I learned that vigorously massaging a man's feet with detailed attention to his toes will enliven him, charge his blood with heat and fire his sexual potency. So chafe your lover's feet between your hands, then rub them well all over, probing deeply with your thumbs into the spaces between the bones. This way you stimulate the energy meridians that lead to the vital organs, and locate many of the sensitive points we use in acupuncture and acupressure, which is also called shiatsu.

'Then hold his foot firmly in one hand, while you work his toes with the other. Pinch along the "seams" of each toe from the root to the tip, then rotate it gently. End by rotating the foot at the ankle. A good foot massage has the miraculous effect of raising the spirits and making the whole body feel "joined-up". You can give yourself a daily foot massage, Adam, to help maintain your overall sexual vitality; even regularly stretching and flexing the feet and toes will help.

'Adam's hands and wrists will benefit from the same treatment,' Koriko told Eve. 'Then give his spine and lower back a massage, pressing down vertically first with your palms, then with your thumbs, working outside the vertebrae from top to bottom. By this time he will be tingling with life and warmth, and feeling the Three Conditions of love we talked about earlier: desire, relaxation and generosity. It is time to work more gently, as you massage and caress the tender skin of his inner arms and legs, which are sensitive erogenous zones.'

'I like to increase the urgency of my lover's desire by indirect means,' said Padmini. 'Try brushing the flat of your palm along the insides of his legs and over his testicles. Do this several times and then continue quickly and lightly up the shaft, hardly touching the tip. Touch the lingam with feather–light fingers as if to draw it up to meet you as you gradually explore its shape. This is an exquisitely tantalizing process for a man, and he will break away from you and renew his ardour in kisses and caresses.

'When you take his lingam in your hand,' she continued, 'be confident, leisurely and firm in all your movements. Give him the feeling that you're completely in control – and in no hurry. Tune in to his needs. Listen to his breathing; watch for in-voluntary movements that tell you how he feels. Tantalize him by changing rhythm or speed and by varying the angle and pressure of your strokes.'

'Some women pump away at the Jade Pillar until their wrists ache,' said Koriko with a giggle. 'But there is no need for boredom or exhaustion! Follow your intuition and your instinct to play. Weigh the Jade Stalk in your hand. Lift it up and let it drop – smack – back onto his belly. Have fun with it. Watch it bounce. Walk your fingers in mischievous steps up the shaft and very lightly tickle the rosy tip as it rises to meet you, or try drumming your fingers on the shaft as if you were playing the flute.'

Marguerite said, 'Hold the shaft firmly in your hand and squeeze repeatedly, first gently and then more vigorously, as you passionately kiss his mouth. Another thing to do while kissing him is to cup his testicles in your hand and gently support and caress them.'

'Yes, that's good,' smiled Padmini, 'it will take his attention away from his lingam and at the same time fire his passion even more. When he can bear it no longer, resume your rhythmic stroking. Eventually his breathing gets more urgent and the movement of his muscles becomes spasmodic. Keep up the pressure and speed, coolly and with control – he needs no distractions now. And when you feel his body tense for the climax, hold on and carry through, not stopping until he subsides.'

'Trust you to gallop away with the story,' said Koriko, laughing. 'Marguerite and I want to talk about delaying ejaculation, not hurrying it along!'

'May I ask,' said Eve hesitantly, 'what to do if Adam loses his erection?'

'Don't take it personally,' said Padmini. 'Don't imagine that your lover is deliberately withholding from you. Women just as much as men need to accept that the lingam is an unreliable organ, and grows more so as a man ages. But of course there are many ways of making love without an erection. You can return to kissing and caressing, or your lover can take the opportunity of paying detailed attention to your yoni. Then again, the lingam doesn't have to be hard to produce pleasure. It has just as many nerve endings soft as it does hard. Indeed, some of my lovers have told me that the pleasure is no different whether they are erect or not. What does take away the pleasure is the pressure to get an erection. So forget the goal of erection and relax. Just as a man can have an erection without an orgasm, he can have an orgasm without an erection, you know.'

This was a fascinating concept and Eve looked

round to catch Adam's eye, but he had wandered off to take a closer look at the Jade Pillar. As he pushed through the scrubby thicket that grew at its base, he saw a man sitting in contemplation between the two gigantic jade balls. He was neither old nor young, he wore a yellow robe and a soft brown hat, and his long mustachios hung down his chest like ropes of liquorice. The stranger rose to his feet and bowed deeply. 'I am Huang–Di,' he announced. 'I have come to share with you the secrets of the Jade Stalk.'

It was none other than the Yellow Emperor of China, who had been dead five thousand years. Adam bowed back and sat down at the Emperor's feet. He was torn between studying the smooth skin and sharp eyes of his immortal teacher, and squint-ing up at the Jade Pillar, which towered so awesomely above them.

'As you can see for yourself, male energy rises,' said the Emperor, 'which is why we Taoists liken it to fire. And we liken female energy to water. In sexual relations it is the job of the fire to bring the water to the boil, and in order to do this it has to keep glowing for a long time without burning itself out. If a man ejaculates before he has satisfied his beloved and falls into an exhausted sleep, his beloved will feel frustrated, whether she voices it or not. Increasing frustration in the bedroom has the habit of spilling over into the rest of life. This is the single most fundamental principle of sexual relations between man and woman. So to help you have a more fulfilling sex life and therefore a happier relationship, I propose to teach you the Yang Secrets of the Jade Bedchamber.'

Adam listened attentively as the Emperor went on, 'Sometimes the Jade Stalk seems to lead a life of its own, yet there are ways in which it can be brought under control. In ancient China we developed certain techniques that immeasurably enhanced sexual pleasure, while at the same time improving our health. We discovered how to delay and even withhold ejaculation so that we could enjoy orgasm after orgasm without losing an erection.'

'How is it possible to have an orgasm without ejaculating?' Adam asked incredulously.

The Emperor smiled. 'It probably comes as a surprise to you to learn that orgasm and ejaculation are two distinct physical processes,' he said. 'Although we in the Orient have known this for thousands of years, your Western scientists worked it out only halfway through the last century. But what they failed to make clear was that – once you understand that orgasm and ejaculation are not the same thing – you can learn to have the orgasm without the ejaculation and keep your erection.

'Let me explain. Orgasm occurs when the prostate and its surrounding tissues powerfully contract, producing the exquisite sensation of climax. Ejaculation, on the other hand, is simply a reflex action that pumps semen through the urethra and out of the Jade Stalk. The orgasm is the height of bliss; the ejaculation is frankly a disappointing experience that leaves a man tired and drained and unable to continue lovemaking. If it happens early on in the lovemaking session, it will be a disappointment for his lover too. And as athletes in your country seem to appreciate, while making love certainly strengthens a man's vital forces, ejaculation always saps his energy. But when a Western man makes love, ejaculation is his goal!' He sighed and shook his head. 'You are missing out, you see, Adam, on a much more exciting and fulfilling erotic experience, in which you can have several orgasms and stay in control.'

'What does it feel like, to have an orgasm without ejaculation?' asked Adam.

'It feels like riding a wave,' said the Emperor, describing one with a graceful movement of his tiny hand. 'Ejaculation is the crashing of the wave onto the beach, but if you avoid it, you will learn to surf the wave and feel intense soaring pleasure, then without losing your erection, let it plateau out and gradually build up to it again. You can keep going like this for as long as you wish, ending in ejaculation if you like, or conserving your energy.'

'Is it something that a Westerner could learn?' asked Adam dubiously.

The Emperor twirled his moustaches. 'All the techniques the courtesans have taught you – the many ways of caressing and kissing, the subtle arts of touching and arousing the woman's Lotus Flower with your fingers and tongue – are both heaven in themselves and ways of prolonging heaven. The path of the Seventh Heaven has deepened your sexual understanding and your pleasure in love; it has already made you slow down and savour each delicious moment. While the courtesans are busy teaching Eve the exotic arts of tantalizing your Jade Pillar, you are ready for your seventh step on the ladder of erotic bliss. I will teach you how to delay ejaculation, so that you can withstand and enjoy Eve's increasingly irresistible skills for as long as possible!

'Now, let me remind you that ejaculation is

nothing more than an involuntary muscle spasm. I will show you how to make it voluntary, so you can control it. To trigger the ejaculation spasm, the nerves need energy and the muscles need blood, and you can learn, by employing various simple physical techniques, to draw the energy and the blood away from the genitals. That's all there is to it, no real mystery, just mastery. Do you see?'

'But how long would it take?' asked Adam.

'You Westerners are always in such a hurry!' said the Emperor. 'The techniques I will teach you need practice to master. Not because they are difficult, but because in the heat of the moment you are likely to forget them. That's why it's best to work at them on your own before you share them with Eve. The practice in itself will be a novel erotic pleasure and increase your knowledge of your own sexuality.

'To learn ejaculation control, you must begin by observing your own arousal very closely. This is always best done alone. There is so much guilt attached to sexual pleasure in the West that most men train themselves, as adolescents, to ejaculate as quickly as they can, to get it over with before they are caught. It's a difficult lesson to unlearn.' The Emperor chuckled. 'In fact the training in fast ejaculation probably began in prehistory, when a man had to make sure he inseminated a woman before he was attacked by a rival; but things have moved on.

'I want you to stroke your Jade Pillar slowly and luxuriously, without embarrassment. Run your hands over your sensitive inner thighs, caress your belly, touch your nipples to see if they react. Explore every delicious sensation. The prostate gland, as I mentioned already, is the epicentre of the orgasm. We call it the Emerald Seat. This treasure is housed at the centre of the pelvis behind the pubic bone and just above the perineum, which you can feel as a wrinkled "seam" of skin between the back of the scrotum and the anus. The prostate gets more sensitive as arousal increases. You can stimulate it through the perineum, as I will tell you in a minute.

'As you fondly stroke your Jade Pillar, I want you to observe that it goes through four stages of arousal: first it lengthens, then it swells; then it grows hard in your hand; and finally, as you continue to stroke it, it generates a fierce and urgent heat. Learn to distinguish these phases one from the other and to recognize how, as you become more excited, all four together lead to that point of no return at which ejaculation becomes inevitable. Maybe you have used this point in the past to develop staying power by thinking of other things, perhaps reciting lists in your head. But true control comes through real understanding and awareness of your arousal, not from ignoring it.

'So now I will teach you five techniques of ejaculation control to be used when your Jade Pillar is long and swollen, hard and hot, and just reaching that exquisite point of no return. Begin by practising them one by one on separate occasions.

'The first technique is *pull down*. Have you noticed that as the climax approaches, your testicles are drawn up more tightly against your body?' Adam nodded. 'Simply draw them back down again. Cup them in your hand, circling the scrotum with thumb and forefinger, and gently pull down. The ejaculation will be delayed.

'The second exercise is *squeeze*. At the point of no return, put the first two fingers of the right hand on the underside of the Jade Stalk just below the glans and the thumb on top, and squeeze. Your urgency will subside.

'Third, *breathe*. You know that your breathing and heart rate accelerate as you approach ejaculation. So it follows that by slowing down your breathing you can delay ejaculation. Start by practising deep breathing when you are not aroused. Place both hands on your lower belly. Inhale and feel the breath push your belly out. Exhale with some force – *huhh!* – pulling the belly back towards your spine and feeling the Jade Stalk and testicles rise up. Then try the exercise when you are aroused. Just before the point of no return, begin deep breathing. The ejaculation will be delayed – maybe not the first time you try it, but keep practising. Remember, losing control of your breathing is losing control.

'The fourth technique is *pump*. As the courtesans have reminded us, there are no muscles in the Jade Pillar. But you can pump the muscles of the pelvic floor to boost the power of your orgasm and strengthen both erection and ejaculation control. The best time to start training is when you urinate. Inhale deeply into your belly, then exhale forcefully while pushing out the urine in a strong stream. Inhale again and contract the pelvic floor to stop the flow of urine in midstream. Repeat the stop–start exercise until you have finished urinating. You may not be able to do it at first, but you will improve with daily practice.

'When you start to make progress, try out your strengthened muscles while you are aroused. Flex the muscles to firm your erection, making the Jade Pillar bob and sway. (Your lover will find this a fascinating sight, by the way!) Then try pumping the muscle hard at the point of no return: your ejaculation will be delayed. Squeezing the pelvic floor muscles around the sperm ducts stops the release of sperm, and pumping the muscle hard draws the blood away from the genitals.'

The Emperor rummaged in the folds of his robe and brought out a small flask and two tiny cups. He uncorked the flask and poured out a steaming brew; Adam caught a whiff of liquorice and ginger. Ginseng was in there too. As they sipped the potent aphrodisiac, Huang–Di said, 'Now for the fifth technique: *push*. You know the perineum is a totally ignored part of the anatomy in the West, but Taoists regard it highly. We call it the Gate of Life and Death. And the point at the middle of the perineum is prized above all others for its role in giving pleasure. Locate it with your finger as a little hollow. This point is so important to Chinese medicine that it has many different names. One of them is Long Strong, because of the amazing effect it has on the

Jade Pillar, and another is the name I love to call it, the Stairway to Heaven.

'When you are fully aroused, push your finger into this point up to the first joint. (This is something you can also get your lover to do for you.) The pressure allows more blood to enter the Jade Sceptre and it will throb with pleasure; hence the name Long Strong. Powerful, rhythmic pressure on the same point imitates the contractions of the prostate, producing an exquisite orgasmic feeling, which is why it is also called the Stairway to Heaven. While you are focused on the pleasure it gives, the urge to ejaculate is interrupted.'

The Emperor tightened the cork in his flask and slipped it back into his robes. 'So now you have five very simple techniques – *pull down*, *squeeze*, *breathe*, *pump* and *push* – to delay ejaculation and prolong lovemaking. The more you practise them, the sooner you will start to experience orgasm without ejaculation – it will happen quite naturally! – and once you have had your first such experience, your enthusiasm for practising will be redoubled.'

Adam smiled. It didn't seem too difficult. 'But if I don't ejaculate, where does the semen go?'

'It is broken down and reabsorbed into the body,' said the Emperor, 'just as sperm are reabsorbed by a man who has had a vasectomy. So the nutrients in the semen that Koriko told you about nourish the body instead of being wasted. Practise these techniques when you can, and find the one that's most effective for you, but don't blame yourself when you forget it right at the last moment. We're not in a race; we're seeking self-knowledge, and that develops slowly. If you manage to master all five techniques, start combining them.'

Adam let out a whistle from between his teeth.

'Yes, it's very tricky, but once you have combined them and added one further technique, the reward is not just orgasm without ejaculation, but an experience you never dreamed was possible for a man – multiple orgasms that you can feel through-out your body! Eventually you will be able to use all six techniques together quite unconsciously, so that you can ride the orgasmic wave.'

Adam said, 'What does it feel like to have a multiple orgasm?'

'You experience a whole range of exquisite sensations. Some are gentle flickering peaks while others are tremendous soaring highs. Some take place in the genitals and others completely submerge you in an orgasm that rolls on and on, lifting you ever higher, like surfing on the biggest wave and never subsiding to wait for the next ride. You become the orgasm. Afterwards you feel brilliant – peaceful, relaxed and full of power. As you can imagine, this is very different from the brief orgasms with ejaculation that you are used to and which leave you exhausted and needing to sleep.'

'Please tell me the sixth technique,' said Adam.

'The sixth technique is *visualizing*. It's an energy exercise (what we call a *chi gung* exercise) that allows you to master the art of drawing your sexual energy from your genitals and circulating it around your body so that your whole body feels orgasmic. Now visualizing is a very advanced technique.

To start with, practise drawing the energy around your body without becoming aroused. First, per-form the pumping technique. As you pull the muscles up, inhale and visualize drawing a glowing ball of sexual energy from the testicles into the perineum and then into the base of the spine. Exhale and pump the muscles down, imagining shooting the ball of sexual energy further up the spine. Continue deep breathing and pumping, visualizing the ball of energy moving right up your back to the top of your head, where it will produce a light tingling sensation. Touch the tip of your tongue to the roof of your mouth. This allows the energy to travel full circuit. Now use deep breath-ing, this time without pumping, as you visualize drawing the ball of energy from the tip of your tongue, and feel it sliding warm and golden like a strong drink, down the front of the body to the belly, pubis and perineum.'

'I think I've got that,' said Adam. 'So I imagine moving a golden ball of hot sexual energy from my genitals up my back, over the top of my head, and down the front of my body, by pumping my pelvic floor muscles and deep breathing?'

'That's right.' Huang twirled his moustaches thoughtfully. 'It sounds strange, I am sure, to Western ears, but this visualization is a very powerful exercise and sometimes a beginner can experience a slight discomfort. If you forget to close the circuit by putting your tongue to the roof of your mouth, for instance, you could get a headache or experience a lot of sneezing, because the energy will be stuck above the mouth. Close the circuit and draw the energy down. If it gets stuck at the front of your body there might be pressure in the solar plexus or stomach. Just keep on visualizing drawing the energy down. If you have uncomfortable pressure in the genitals, use deep breathing, pump the pelvic floor muscles or allow yourself to ejaculate to release the pressure.

'Now here is how we pull all the strands together to experience riding the orgasmic wave. Begin by stroking your Jade Pillar and when you reach the point of no return, stop and breathe deeply to get control. Hold your breath for several seconds until the urge to ejaculate subsides. Pump the pelvic floor muscle around the prostate, which is on the point of contracting and will feel very sensitive.

'Now use the three hand techniques I've just taught you one after the other, pausing after each to gain control by deep breathing and pumping. First squeeze the Jade Stalk with your fingers and thumb. When you have regained control, push your finger hard into the Stairway to Heaven. This refocuses your attention and interrupts the ejaculation reflex. Release and pull down the scrotum. Finally, visualize drawing the fiery ball of sexual energy away from the genitals and around the body.

'The urge to ejaculate will have passed and you will relax into the heavenly experience of surfing the orgasmic wave with its many ecstatic whole-body sensations.'

'Sounds good, but that's a lot to remember!' said Adam. He was secretly wondering if his erection would be strong enough to withstand the six techniques all at once.

The Emperor chuckled. 'As I told you, combining all six techniques is a very advanced practice. You may never get that far, but the more you work at each individual technique, especially the first five, the more instinctive they'll become. Orgasms will just start to happen, and your erection will still be there. Then they'll get stronger, more explosive, and still your Jade Pillar will stand firm. It's a thrilling voyage of sexual self-discovery. And there will be times when you lose your erection altogether. But if you continue to practise you might discover something else surprising. It's quite possible to have an orgasm without erection, you know!'

The Emperor could read his mind! Adam thanked him with a deep bow.

'There is only one further thing I need to tell you,' said Huang, 'but it is most important. These exercises are just techniques, no more than that. They will help you to greater self-knowledge and self-mastery and allow you to experience a new kind of pleasure. But they are not love. So when you practise them with Eve, do so in a spirit of humility and loving kindness, not with arrogance or boastfulness. As your sexual confidence increases, you will in any case be able to let go of all egotistical behaviour and the insecurity that prompts it.'

These last crucial words were uttered in something of a hurry. There was a sudden sucking noise – *'thweeet'* – like a sharp intake of breath crossed with the popping of a cork, and the Emperor spiralled upwards in a wisp of mist and vanished in the direction of Beijing. Adam, standing alone at the base of the awesome Jade Pillar, looked about himself, bemused.

While Adam was being initiated into the Yang Secrets of the Jade Bedchamber by the Yellow Emperor of China, the courtesans were discussing with Eve the many imaginative ways of pleasuring a man without putting the Jade Stalk inside the Cinnabar Cleft.

Padmini suggested massaging the lingam between the breasts, generously lubricated with almond oil, a fine oil with a delicate nutty taste that interferes little with the natural aromas of skin and sexual secretions. 'If Adam sits in a comfortable chair, then you can kneel between his legs,' she told Eve. 'Stroke his lingam with your hands to work in the oil, which is in itself a luxurious experience. Hold the root of the lingam with one hand and squeeze your breasts together around it with the other. Slide it slowly up and down in your cleavage by moving your hips as if you were riding a horse, sometimes pushing the tip of the lingam up as far as your tongue. You can refocus his attention and

change the pace by releasing the lingam and swinging your breasts against it; drag them voluptuously
across it and tickle the rosy head with your nipples.'

'Some women are not as well endowed as Eve,'
said Marguerite, cupping her own small breasts in
her hands – they were as shallow and pert as
champagne glasses. 'But when my lover is lying
down I can rub my breasts over his Ivory Spear as
I gyrate my body above him. This massage is a
deliciously sensual experience for both lovers;
when he is only partly erect it feels less deliberate
and demanding than touching with the hands.'

Padmini was eager to tell them how 'Sucking the
Mango' was performed in classical India. 'Educated
courtesans knew that Sucking the Mango was the
ultimate experience of bliss for a man,' she said.
'Kings and princes and ministers of state all gave
lavish gifts of jewels and property to experience the
most sophisticated forms of the art. Men who
couldn't afford to keep a courtesan, employed
servants to do it for them – they were called

euphemistically "shampooers", which meant masseurs. The women of the harem, of course, secretly practised the arts of the tongue on each other or on the eunuchs who were supposed to be guarding them; many of our eunuchs were capable of handsome erections . . .

'Eunuchs also worked in massage parlours disguised as women to give sexual favours to their male customers', she confided. 'Of course, the client knew that he was being massaged by a man, but it was never acknowledged, and this gave him the secret thrill of indulging in a forbidden delight. Let us imagine it went something like this. After a thorough all-over body massage, when the client was relaxed and tingling with well-being, the eunuch would pay careful and delicate attention to his upper thighs and abdomen. This was the start of a little game between them, which always had the same erotic outcome. When the man's lingam responded to the tantalizing massage, the eunuch would take it in his hands, chiding his client for getting into such a state, and stroke it, pretending that this would calm the man's inappropriate lust. If the man said nothing, the eunuch would continue stroking and chiding until the lingam was so hard and hot that it was aching to be sucked; but if the man ordered him to suck it, he would protest, and pretend to give in only reluctantly.

'Eventually he took the man's lingam between his lips, and moved it this way and that. Sometimes he thrust it more deeply inside his mouth and pulled it right out again, uttering a little sigh and tickling the tip with his tongue before continuing to thrust. At other times, he would move the lingam from side to side, every so often letting it plop out of his mouth, then sucking it back in again, or coaxing it back in with his tongue. From time to time, the eunuch would tease his client by complaining of tiredness and expressing a wish to stop, but of course the client would always ask, then angrily command, then fervently entreat him to continue.

'The next stage was to drive the man wild with

more reticent stimulation. This is a very good tactic – if your lover feels you are deliberately not doing quite enough to stimulate him, it makes his excitement more urgent than ever. So the eunuch covered the end of his master's lingam modestly with his fingers pressed together like a lotus bud, and delicately licked and nibbled at the shaft. Then, when the man kept moaning for more and his agony for release was intolerable, his servant gave in and sucked at the head of the lingam, gradually taking it further and further into his mouth in a vigorous action that entirely accorded with his master's wishes. Finally, the man could bear it no longer and implored his servant to rush to the finale, which was called "swallowing up"!'

'And what about swallowing?' asked Eve doubtfully. 'Do I have to do it?'

'When you play at Sucking the Mango, you must be in control all the way,' said Padmini, 'so let your lover know that he should not move his hips to thrust, unless, of course, you want him to. Then the decision of how deeply to take the lingam into your mouth and whether to swallow is up to you. If you haven't ever swallowed semen before, take some on the tip of your finger and try it. It feels warm and may taste delightfully nutty, salty or sweet. The taste is directly affected by your lover's health and by what he has been eating and drinking. If you like it, the sexiest way to swallow it is to drink it down greedily immediately on ejaculation. (Remember, there is no more than a teaspoonful.) Some men like their lovers to carry on licking and sucking through the several spasms of their ejaculation – it makes them feel as though their ejaculation is never–ending – but with others the glans becomes so sensitive that after the first spasm they can no longer bear to be touched. To kiss him afterwards with the taste of his semen in your mouth is a sensational erotic delight.'

'In the West complicated feelings of guilt and rejection sometimes surround the art of swallowing,' said Marguerite. 'Some women feel they should do it to prove the strength of their love, while others feel that if their lover really cared for them, he wouldn't want to ejaculate in their mouth. In fact it is simply a matter of what you like, and not to be seen as a proof of love. Far more important than swallowing is being honest about your feelings on the subject. It may be that Adam decides to practise the art of withholding ejaculation as you suck him. It may be that as you feel his body tense and spasm, you withdraw the Ivory Spear from your mouth and let its pearls drop around your neck, which explains the meaning of the delightful love term "pearl necklace". Or you could let them shoot warmly onto your closed lips and fingertips and massage them into the still throbbing Spear until it subsides, or into your own skin. Be imaginative, be playful, and above all, be free!'

'For me,' said Padmini warmly, 'Sucking the Mango is the ultimate intimacy, the ultimate devotion. Making love in this way, you can really study and adore your lover's secret anatomy. You can know it better than he knows it himself. Some men love to have their testicles sucked and licked too. But I prefer to just cup them in my hand and watch the way the skin moves over them – like rippling waves on the surface of the sea.'

'Padmini, how poetic!' said Eve. 'Tell me, how do you feel about sixty–nine, where the lovers lick each other?'

'*Soixante-neuf* is very overrated,' said Marguerite. 'Trying to concentrate on two things at once doesn't allow you to relax and succumb to the sensuality of either sensation. If you like to lie in the head–to–tail position, tell your lover that he is not allowed to touch, but only to look, because you want him to lose himself in the delicious sensations of being sucked.'

Eve said, 'How do I avoid getting tired? I find keeping my mouth wide open for a long time uncomfortable. And how do I avoid biting him?'

'The Latin term *fellatio* means "suck",' said Marguerite. 'Sucking and licking are exquisite pleasures for both partners; fellatio need not involve any deep throat techniques. But before it stands erect, it's easy to take the Ivory Spear completely inside your mouth. This is a beautifully sensitive and warming way to arouse passion in your lover.'

'Once he is fully aroused,' said Padmini, 'you can suck the glans for a long time without tiring. You can nuzzle the shaft of the lingam with the warm wet insides of your lips and apply pressure with the flat of your tongue as your mouth moves up and down towards the tip. First one side and then the other. Let it fall out of your mouth with a slurp and press your cheeks and your face against it, as if you can't get enough of it. Lean above his body and work the top, licking with the flat of your tongue right from the root to the tip in a big sweeping movement. Be energetic and thorough!'

'If you practise licking, sucking the tip and sliding the open lips along the shaft,' said Marguerite, 'you won't be in any danger of hurting him with your teeth, though some men do like gentle, teasing nibbles.'

Padmini said, 'A mixture of hand work and mouth work is pure heaven for a man. Hold the lingam in your hand and lubricate it well, drenching it with saliva or almond oil. Then work it very slowly and deliberately up and down in your fist, all the while lavishly licking the head. Make greedy sucking noises and produce lots of saliva, moving your hand lightly and rapidly up and down the shaft and tickling the opening of the urethra with the tip of your tongue. Accelerate to light, well-lubricated and flowing movements, letting your mouth follow your hand in a hypnotic rhythm, so he hardly knows where the sensation is coming from.'

❦

'And now listen to the Secrets of the Jade Boudoir,' said Koriko. 'They will teach you how to become a tigress in the bedroom. Why do you think geishas whiten their faces and put high spots of rouge on their cheeks? Because it suggests a fevered imagination within their perfect composure that men find extremely erotic. So remember this when you sit in front of your mirror, but don't exaggerate the eroticism of your appearance in any way, for he must not suspect you are conscious of it. Let him think it is his secret alone. Have you noticed the way geishas paint small rosebud lips in the centre of their mouths? Have you ever wondered why? They make their mouths look smaller so the Jade Stalk looks bigger when they are Playing the Flute.

'When you make love to your Jade Prince, don't undress', she said, 'but just expose part of your body – your breasts, say – to heighten his desire and imagination and keep the connection with the everyday that is so important for your own sexual satisfaction. Thus he will look at you during the day with more longing. He will also love the feel of urgency and inflamed passion suggested by partial undress. He should not undress either. If he attempts to take off his clothes, stop him. Simply loosen his shirt and pants and take out his Jade Stalk. It is sure to be inflamed already by the bold submissiveness of your approach.

'Don't allow him to lie down while you Play the Flute, because for a woman to bend over a man who is lying suggests that she is in control. He should either stand or sit. To heighten his fantasy of submission, you must kneel in front of him. Avoid squatting, as this is the position women use to urinate and defecate and it will send the wrong subconscious message. To give him the most intense sensual experience, make sure he can see his Jade Stalk in your mouth. Positioning yourself so he can see will also mean that his Jade Stalk is pulled downwards slightly, trapping more blood in the head and shaft and thereby increasing his sexual energy and his orgasm.

'Produce as much saliva as you can during the encounter. It will excite your Jade Prince to see saliva drooling and gushing from your lips around his Jade Stalk. It will seem in his imagination that his ejaculate is never-ending, pumping on and on. Increase his ardour still further by making noises. Not only loud sucking and slurping sounds, but little sighs and low trembling groans. Let the sounds come out quite naturally – don't be theatrical or he will suspect you are insincere and his fantasy will be shattered.

'Have him place a hand on the back of your neck or the top of the head as you lick and suck to give him a sure sense of his own power. But if he starts to exert pressure with his hand, ask him softly to be gentle. Never say you dislike anything. Always be positive, exciting and playful. Never be crude.

'Geishas do not often swallow semen. We value it too much for its special properties as a skin cream! So when the precious hot essence squirts from the Jade Stalk, tilt back your head and let him see it come onto your neck or breasts. Then rub the pearl necklace he has given you lasciviously into your skin. You need not tell him you are doing this to rejuvenate your complexion, eliminate wrinkles and prevent age spots!

'Playing the Flute is a wonderful exercise to tone all the facial muscles and strengthen the gums. It also encourages deep breathing through the nose and strengthens the lungs. I have mentioned the importance of creating as much saliva as possible. Saliva is full of nutrients, it aids digestion, heals the skin, keeps the teeth and gums in peak condition, pink and firm, and when you do gulp it down, it cleans the oesophagus. All this will help keep you young.

'Now, I often give my students a little exercise in concentration that helps with Playing the Flute. It is to take a raisin in your mouth. Suck on it until it dissolves. It will take a long time. Think of nothing but the raisin. Learn not only its taste, but its texture. Completely lose yourself in appreciating that raisin until you *become* it. This is a useful exercise in surrender and communication that will improve your Flute Playing.

'On another occasion you might prefer not to Play the Flute, but to stroke the Jade Stalk with your hand until your Prince reaches orgasm. Use oil lavishly to make it excitingly slick. For this exercise too, you should kneel before your Jade Prince and bare your breasts. Pull the Jade Stalk down towards you so it hardens more quickly and appears longer as he gazes down on it, and though you don't intend to mouth it, open your mouth and stick out your tongue towards its tip, again so that he can watch. Gently flick your tongue in time with your hand movements. I can guarantee he will find it unbearably erotic.'

Koriko bowed. The fascinating lesson was over. Eve returned the bow deeply, her eyes sparkling and her cheeks flushed with excitement. She was about to express her amazement and her gratitude when they caught sight of Adam, returning from his conversation with the Emperor.

'What you should do now, Eve,' Koriko whispered, taking her by the hand, 'is forget everything we have taught you and know only one thing, that every act of love is not technique, not artifice, nor even skill, but a simple human ceremony of the heart.'

EPILOGUE

The Seventh Heaven

Continue to explore the path of the Seventh Heaven, to use its arts as the bedrock of your intimate life, and to inspire you to treat sex with curiosity and reverence.

ADAM AND EVE HAD COME TO THE end of their fascinating journey. They had studied the seven scrolls and practised the ancient wisdom that they taught. Now in a beautiful garden, where birds sang and monkeys chattered, they met to bid farewell to the three courtesans who had been their guides.

'On your erotic journey you have explored seven aspects of love,' said Koriko, as they sat together in the shade of a blooming kadamba tree. 'You studied them separately in order to deepen your under-standing of each in turn. But now let us blur the seven into one. For in the realm of the erotic, technique means nothing compared to an attitude of complete awareness and relaxed openness to experience, sensual and spiritual.

'The greatest sexual power that you have resides in your mind. Be sure to use it. When your intention is profound, so the feelings you transmit in your kisses and caresses will speak profoundly of the desires of your heart.'

'Inside this pavilion,' said Marguerite, pointing to a little house almost hidden among the trees, 'a bed awaits you, festooned with garlands of flowers and spread with a fresh white coverlet. It is your marriage bed. A feast is laid out to welcome you, with cooling fruits, and wine. After your period of abstinence, you will come together charged with erotic excitement as on the first night you spent in each other's arms, but with more confidence, deeper desire, and slower, more lasting pleasure.

'And so the end of your erotic journey is but the last step before the beginning, for you are about to discover that the knowledge of the seven scrolls has transformed your lovemaking. You have practised many imaginative ways of expressing erotic love without breaking your vow of abstinence. Continue to explore the path of the Seventh Heaven, to use its arts as the bedrock of your intimate life, and to inspire you to treat sex with curiosity and reverence.'

'You have taken the seven steps and passed through the seven gateways,' said Padmini, 'and now it is time to look back and contemplate all you have learned, and then to forget, and to allow love to flow naturally, instinctively. For as we told you once before, "When the wheel of ecstasy is in full motion, there is no textbook at all, and no order."'

ACKNOWLEDGEMENTS

Many, many thanks to my far-sighted and judicious editor, Brenda Kimber, who sees both what is there and what is not. Thanks to her team at Bantam: editor Nicky Jeanes for her enthusiasm, copy editor Beth Humphries for her eye for detail, and designers Fiona Andreanelli for the elegant layout, and Paul Gooney for capturing the spirit of the book in his striking cover.

Three friends need a special mention. Philippa Bridges, for her kindness, and for our long walks, when we talked of other things. Noëlle Francis for her thorough understanding of the creative mire, and for being a willing sounding-board. And Cindy Engel for practical suggestions and a sense of humour that by recognizing the enormity of obstacles, somehow cuts them neatly down to size. Caroline Davidson is truly my No. 1 Ladies' Literary Agent. Thank you, Caroline, for your inspiring personality, your surprising and ingenious mind, and the many laughs we have shared.

Finally, I want to thank my wonderful teachers at the Norwich College of Shiatsu, who have had nothing and everything to do with my progress through this book.

GLOSSARY

Chakra Energy centre, literally 'wheel'. There are seven vortices of energy along the spine. They correspond to the endocrine glands and resonate with different vibrations of sound and colour, different symbols, scents and emotions. The chakras are used in the practice of Tantra and the Tao to gain mystic enlightenment through meditation.

Chi The universal energy or life force. See Taoism, yin and yang.

Cinnabar Cave Vulva.

Cinnabar Cleft The rima, the cleft between the two outer lips of the vulva.

Cinnabar Field Female genitals.

Cinnabar Gate Vaginal opening.

Cock's Crest The penis.

Coral Grotto The vulva.

Courtly Love The erotic religion of medieval Europe. It had its roots in Tantra and its heart at the court of Queen Eleanor of Aquitaine in Poitiers. Courtly Love was invariably secret and adulterous.

Diamond, Diamond Seat The clitoris.

Divine Field   The exquisitely sensitive area above the clitoris.

Emerald Seat   The prostate.

Floating World   The pleasure quarter of Edo, the old city of Tokyo.

Frenulum   In a man, the wrinkled skin at the point where the foreskin is attached to the glans of the penis. In a woman, the same point on the clitoris.

Garland of Happiness   The corona – the fleshy lip that runs like a collar beneath the head of the penis.

Gate of Life and Death   The perineum.

Geisha   An artist of life, the most elusive erotic icon of the East.

Golden Gulley   The upper part of the vulva.

Golden Lotus   The vulva.

Golden Spring   Female urethral opening.

Golden Vase   The vagina.

Heavenly Dragon Pillar   The penis.

Heavenly Wings   The hood or tent under which the clitoris withdraws.

Hidden Place   The vagina.

High Tide   Female orgasm.

Ivory Spear   The penis.

Jade Balls   The testicles.

Jade Fountain   The vulva.

Jade Gate   In a woman, the vaginal opening. In a man, the meatus, the opening at the tip of the penis.

Jade Pillar   The penis.

Jade Pouch   The scrotum.

Jade Sceptre   The penis.

Jade Stalk   The penis.

Jade Vein   The lower part of the vulva.

Jambu, Paradise Island of   The vulva.

Kama   Everything that delights the senses.

Kundalini   The slumbering serpent of energy that lies coiled around the lower two chakras. Meditation causes it to rise up the spine.

Lingam   The penis – literally 'wand of light'.

Long Strong   The midpoint of the perineum, a powerful point in acupuncture and the sexual practices of the East.

Lotus   The vulva.

Lotus-eating   Cunnilingus, licking the vulva.

Lute Strings   The frenulum of the glans penis or clitoris. (See Frenulum).

Moon blood   Menstrual blood.

Open Peony Blossom   The vulva.

Perineum   The muscular bridge between the genitals and the anus, central to all Eastern spiritual and sexual practice.

Playing the Flute   Fellatio, sucking the penis.

Red Bird   The penis.

Red Petals   The inner lips of the vulva, the labia minora.

Rima   The cleft between the outer lips of the vulva (labia majora).

Stairway to Heaven   The midpoint of the perineum, a powerful point in acupuncture and the sexual practices of the East.

Sucking the Mango   Fellatio, sucking the penis.

Swelling Mushroom   The penis.

Tantra   An Eastern discipline that marries spirituality and sexuality. Its basic principle is that women possess more spiritual and sexual energy than men, who become sexually exhausted relatively quickly. Its aim is to find ways of prolonging sexual activity without exhaustion, to the benefit of both sexes. Its essence is an attitude of complete openness and awareness, both spiritual and sexual.

Taoism   A worldview originating in China. The Tao (pronounced 'Dow') is 'The Way'. At the heart of Taoism is the idea of a universal life force or energy called chi. The aim of Taoism is to maximize the flow of chi in the body and to use its transformational power for physical and spiritual health.

Three Fountains   Sources of the precious yin essence in a woman's body: the Red Lotus Fountain of the lips, the Twin Lotus Fountains of the breasts, and the Purple Agaric Fountain of the yoni.

Tree of Life   The shaft of the penis.

Turtle's Head   The head or glans of the penis.

Vajra   The penis – literally 'tool of consciousness'.

Vajrasana   The clitoris.

Velvet head   The head or glans of the penis.

Yin and yang The two opposing principles that create chi, the life force. Yin is passive, while yang is active – they capture and release each other like the two halves of a circle, refreshing and renewing the life force they generate between them. One of the many ways of bringing yin and yang into harmony is through sex.

Yoni The vulva – literally 'sacred place'.

BIBLIOGRAPHY

Allende, Isabel, *Aphrodite: The Love of Food and the Food of Love*, Flamingo, 1998.

Al-Rawi, Rosina-Fawzia, *Grandmother's Secrets: The Ancient Rituals and Healing Power of Belly Dancing*, trans. Monique Arav, Interlink Books, 1999.

Andreae, Simon, *The Secrets of Love & Lust*, Abacus, 2000.

Bayley, Stephen, ed., *Sex*, Cassell, 2001.

Bechtel, Stefan, Laurence Roy Stains and the editors of *Men's Health* Books, *Sex: A Man's Guide*, Rodal Press, 1996.

Bhattacharji, Sukumari, 'Prostitution in Ancient India', from *Women in Early Indian Societies*, ed. Roy Kumkum, Manohar, 1999.

Blue, Adrianne, *On Kissing*, Victor Gollancz, 1996.

Bornoff, Nicholas, *Pink Samurai, An Erotic Exploration of Japanese Society*, Grafton, 1991.

Brazell, Karen, trans., *The Confessions of Lady Nijo*, Peter Owen, 1975.

Burns, E. Jane, *Courtly Love Undressed: Reading through Clothes in Medieval French Literature*, University of Pennsylvania Press, 2002.

Burton, Richard and F.F. Arbuthnot, trans., *The Perfumed Garden of Sheikh Nefzawi*, HarperCollins, 1993.

Burton, Richard and F.F. Arbuthnot, trans., *The Illustrated Kama Sutra, Ananga Ranga, Perfumed Garden*, Hamlyn, 1987.

Capellanus, Andreas, *The Art of Courtly Love*, trans. John Jay Parry, Columbia University Press, 1960.

Chang, Jolan, *The Tao of Love & Sex*, Wildwood House, 1977.

Chevalier, Jean and Alain Gheerbrant, *The Penguin Dictionary of Symbols*, trans. John Buchanan–Brown, Penguin Books, 1996.

Chia, Mantak and Douglas Abrams, *The Multi-Orgasmic Man: Sexual Secrets That Every Man Should Know*, Thorsons, 2002.

Chu, Valentin, *The Yin-Yang Butterfly. Ancient Chinese*

Sexual Secrets for Western Lovers, Simon & Schuster, 1994.

Dalby, Liza, *Geisha*, University of California Press, 1998.

Deng, Ming–Dao, *Chronicles of Tao*, HarperSanFrancisco, 1993.

Doniger, Wendy and Sudhir Kakar, trans., *Kamasutra* by Vatsyayana Mallanaga, Oxford University Press, 2002.

Epton, Nina, *Love and the French*, Cassell, 1959.

Frayling, Christopher, *Vampyres*, Faber & Faber, 1991.

Friedman, David M., *A Mind of Its Own. A Cultural History of the Penis*, The Free Press, 2001.

Gies, Joseph and Frances, *Life in a Medieval City*, Arthur Barker, 1969.

Glass, Lillian, *He Says, She Says. Closing the Communication Gap between the Sexes*, Piatkus, 1992.

Hecker, H–U., A. Steveling, E. Peuker, J. Kastner and K. Liebchen, *Color Atlas of Acupuncture*, Thieme, 1999.

Hite, Shere, *The Hite Report*, Macmillan, 1976.

Hite, Shere, *The Hite Report on Male Sexuality*, Optima, 1978.

Johari, Harish, *Ayurvedic Massage. Traditional Indian Techniques for Balancing Body and Mind*, Healing Arts Press, 1996.

Jones, Alison, *Larousse Dictionary of World Folklore*, Larousse, 1995.

Lai, Hsi, *The Sexual Teachings of the White Tigress: Secrets of the Female Taoist Masters*, Destiny Books, 2001.

Leclercq, Geho and Sarita Newman, *Tantric Love: Journey into Sexual and Spiritual Ecstasy*, Gaia Books, 2001.

Markale, Jean, *Courtly Love: The Path of Sexual Initiation*, trans. Jon Graham, Inner Traditions, 2000.

Marlis, Stefanie, *The Art of the Bath*, Chronicle Books, 1997.

Marshall, Fiona, *Natural Aphrodisiacs*, Element Books, 2000.

Mills, Jane, *Sexwords*, Penguin Books, 1993.

Montagu, Ashley, *Touching: The Human Significance of the Skin*, Harper & Row, 1971.

Morris, Desmond, *Bodywatching*, HarperCollins, 1985.

Morris, Ivan, trans., *The Pillow Book of Sei Shonagon*, Penguin Classics, 1971.

Opie, Iona and Moira Tatem, *A Dictionary of Superstitions*, Oxford University Press, 1992.

Ovid, *The Art of Love*, trans. James Michie, Random House, 2002.

Paley, Maggie, *The Book of the Penis*, Grove Press, 1999.

Payne, Peter, *Martial Arts: The Spiritual Dimension*, Thames & Hudson, 1981.

Phillips, Adam, *On Kissing, Tickling and Being Bored*, Harvard University Press, 1993.

Ramesh, Gita, *Ayurvedic Herbal Massage*, Roli Books, 2000.

Reid, Daniel P., *The Tao of Health, Sex, & Longevity*, Simon & Schuster, 1989.

Rich, Penny, *Pamper Your Partner*, Hamlyn, 1990.

Russell, Stephen and Jürgen Kolb, *The Tao of Sexual Massage*, Gaia Books, 1992.

Sampson, Val, *Tantra, The Art of Mind-Blowing Sex*, Vermilion, 2002.

Silver, Burton and Heather Busch, *Kokigami: Performance-enhancing Adornments for the Adventurous Man*, Ten Speed Press, 2000.

Singh, Sarva Daman, 'Polyandry in the Vedic Period', from *Women in Early Indian Societies*, ed. Roy Kumkum, Manohar, 1999.

Sinha, Indra, *Tantra, The Cult of Ecstasy*, Hamlyn, 1993.

Smith, Bruce and Yoshiko Yamamoto, *The Japanese Bath*, Gibbs Smith, 2001.

Sonntag, Linda, *The Photographic Kamasutra*, Hamlyn, 2001.

Spiegel, Maura and Lithe Sebesta, *The Breast Book: Attitude, Perception, Envy and Etiquette*, Workman Publishing, 2002.

Stubbs, Kenneth Ray, *Erotic Passions: A Guide to Orgasmic Massage, Sensual Bathing, Oral Pleasuring, and Ancient Sexual Positions*, Secret Garden Publishing, 2000.

Taberner, Peter V., *Aphrodisiacs. The Science and the Myth*, Croom Helm, 1985.

Tanizaki, Junichiro, *In Praise of Shadows*, Vintage Classic, 2001.

Tannahill, Reay, *Sex in History*, Hamish Hamilton, 1980.

Tannen, Deborah, *You Just Don't Understand: Women and Men in Conversation*, Virago, 1991.

Taylor, Timothy, *The Prehistory of Sex: Four Million Years of Human Sexual Culture*, Fourth Estate, 1996.

Turner, E.S., *A History of Courting*, Michael Joseph, 1954.

Walker, Barbara, *The Woman's Dictionary of Symbols and Sacred Objects*, HarperCollins, 1998.

Walker, Barbara, *The Women's Encyclopedia of Myths and Secrets*, Castle Books, 1996.

Walters, Cecilia, *Geisha Secrets: A Pillow Book for Lovers*, Eddison Sadd Editions, 2000.

Watson, Lyall, *Jacobson's Organ and the Remarkable Nature of Smell*, Allen Lane The Penguin Press, 1999.

Willy, A., L. Vander and O. Fisher, Drs, *The Encyclopaedia of Sex Practice*, London Encyclopaedic Press, 1933.

Wilson, Glenn D. and Chris McLaughlin, *The Science of Love*, Fusion Press, 2001.

Yalom, Marilyn, *A History of the Breast*, Pandora, 1998.

Young, Lailan, *Love around the World*, Hodder & Stoughton, 1985.

Zilbergeld, Bernie, *The New Male Sexuality*, Bantam Books, 1992.

Linda Sonntag is the author of a number of books on sexuality – including the international bestseller *The Photographic Kama Sutra*. She is a qualified shiatsu practitioner. She lives in Suffolk.

INDEX

Page numbers in bold refer to entries in the Glossary.